W9-AMV-062

AUG -- 2018

THE
AUTOIMMUNE
SOLUTION
COOKBOOK

Also by Amy Myers, MD

The Autoimmune Solution

The Thyroid Connection

THE AUTOIMMUNE SOLUTION COOKBOOK

OVER 150 DELICIOUS RECIPES *to* PREVENT *and* REVERSE *the* FULL SPECTRUM *of* INFLAMMATORY SYMPTOMS *and* DISEASES

AMY MYERS, MD

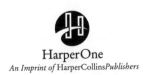

HarperOne
An Imprint of HarperCollinsPublishers

HarperOne

Family photographs by Ziem Malkani

Food photographs by Jennifer Davick

The following are registered or unregistered trademarks of Amy Myers: Amy Myers MD®, The Myers Way®, Get to the root. Learn the tools. Live the Solution®, Candifense™, Microb-Clear™, Primal Earth Probiotic™, Candida Breakthrough™, Leaky Gut Breakthrough™, Parasite Breakthrough™, and Methylation Support™. All rights reserved.

This book contains advice and information relating to health care. It should be used to supplement rather than replace the advice of your doctor or another trained health professional. If you know or suspect you have a health problem, it is recommended that you seek your physician's advice before embarking on any medical program or treatment. All efforts have been made to assure the accuracy of the information contained in this book as of the date of publication. This publisher and the author disclaim liability for any medical outcomes that may occur as a result of applying the methods suggested in this book.

THE AUTOIMMUNE SOLUTION COOKBOOK. Copyright © 2018 by Amy Myers, MD. All rights reserved. Printed in the United States of America. No part of this book may be used or reproduced in any manner whatsoever without written permission except in the case of brief quotations embodied in critical articles and reviews. For information, address HarperCollins Publishers, 195 Broadway, New York, NY 10007.

HarperCollins books may be purchased for educational, business, or sales promotional use. For information, please email the Special Markets Department at SPsales@harpercollins.com.

FIRST EDITION

Designed by SBI Book Arts, LLC

Library of Congress Cataloging-in-Publication Data

Names: Myers, Amy (Physician) author.
Title: The autoimmune solution cookbook : over 150 delicious recipes to prevent and reverse the full spectrum of inflammatory symptoms and diseases / Amy Myers, MD
Description: First edition. | New York, NY : HarperOne, [2018]
Identifiers: LCCN 2018010173 | ISBN 9780062853547 (hardback)
Subjects: LCSH: Autoimmune diseases—Diet therapy—Recipes. | BISAC: HEALTH & FITNESS / Diseases / Immune System. | COOKING / Health & Healing / LCGFT: Cookbooks.
Classification: LCC RC600 .M942 2018 | DDC 641.5/631—dc23 LC record available at https://lccn.loc.gov/2018010173

18 19 20 21 22 LSC(H) 10 9 8 7 6 5 4

To

MOM AND DAD

*For teaching me how to bake and cook
and for instilling in me the importance of a
nourishing diet and real whole food.*

AND MY DAUGHTER, ELLE

*You are my everything.
I can't wait to bake and cook with you.*

Contents

Introduction . . . 1

Part One
Live the Solution

1. My Journey . . . 13

   The Myers Way Symptom Tracker . . . 19

2. The Four Pillars of The Myers Way® . . . 23

Part Two
Ingredients and Kitchen Tools

3. What You Need in Your Kitchen . . . 39

   Foods to Enjoy . . . 74

   Foods to Toss . . . 77

Part Three
Nourishing You and Your Family

4. Breakfast . . . 87

5. Smoothies, Juices, and Other Beverages . . . 103

6. Soups and Salads . . . 133

7. Main Courses ... 151

8. Sides ... 181

9. Dressings, Sauces, and Condiments ... 195

10. Snacks ... 213

11. Desserts ... 227

    Specific Diet Chart ... 247

12. Home and Body ... 257

Part Four

The Myers Way® for Life

13. Getting the Whole Family on Board ... 267

14. Travel Tips ... 273

15. Dining Out ... 275

16. Sleep ... 279

17. Food Reintroduction ... 283

18. Supplements ... 289

Acknowledgments ... 297
Resources ... 299
Index ... 309
About the Author ... 325

Introduction

When Debra first came to see me, she was so sick with autoimmune-related symptoms that she had to rely on a wheelchair to get around. She struggled to wake up in the morning, and by mid-afternoon she was exhausted. She had tried just about everything conventional medicine had to offer her and she was desperate for a solution to her symptoms. However, in all of her many visits to doctors, including numerous specialists, not one medical professional recommended that she focus on the food she was eating as part of her treatment.

I talked to Debra about a natural approach to reversing her condition and explained that food had both the power to harm *and* the power to heal. I developed a treatment plan for Debra that focused on optimizing her diet with real, whole foods that were rich in the nutrients her body needed to heal while avoiding the toxic and inflammatory foods that were making her sick. We also looked at other factors that were contributing to her symptoms, including gut health, toxins, infections, and stress, and devised a plan to address each of those. Within six months of the first time Debra came to see me, she walked into my office, no wheelchair in sight. Not only that, all of her symptoms had fully reversed. Debra said she hadn't felt this good in decades and woke up every day with tremendous energy.

Stories like Debra's are what drive me to do what I do every day because I, too, have been sick and hopeless while dealing with an autoimmune condition. Just like so many of you, my conventional doctors never looked for the root causes of my condition, much less told me that my autoimmunity could be reversed through diet and lifestyle changes. Conventional medicine failed me, and it is my mission to not let it fail you too. I opened my functional medicine clinic to provide patients with the comprehensive approach that I never received from my doctors. Then, wanting to empower even more people, I wrote my *New York Times* bestselling book, *The Autoimmune Solution,* so that people all over the world could experience life-changing results, just like Debra.

Since *The Autoimmune Solution* was released, I have received amazing accounts of radical healing from tens of thousands of you who have used The Myers Way® thirty-day protocol. Thank you so much for your inspiration! Your successes mean the world to me, and your commitment to taking back your health and the health of your families motivates me every day to continue my mission.

Let's catch up quickly on what's been going on in my life since *The Autoimmune Solution* was published. For a long time, my health was not just stable—it was optimal. I felt like I was in the prime of my life. I had a successful and thriving medical practice where people flew from around the world to see me. I was regularly appearing on *The Dr. Oz Show.* I had traveled to India, South America, and Central America. And I had married the man of my dreams. I was at the healthiest point of what I call the autoimmune spectrum (page 21).

Because I was feeling great and all of my autoimmune markers were negative, I did what I have many of my patients do: I added more variety into my diet. Now don't get me wrong; I didn't go crazy and start eating gluten or dairy, however I did reintroduce some of the foods that I knew I could tolerate in moderation. This meant that when I went to India, I ate rice and legumes, and while vacationing with my husband, I sometimes ordered scrambled eggs at breakfast. And because I was traveling more, I was eating out more, which meant that I was sometimes eating foods that were not 100 percent certified organic. And I was enjoying a gluten-free and dairy-free dessert on occasion.

Then, just as I was about to submit the manuscript for my second *New York Times* bestselling book, *The Thyroid Connection,* I became really, really sick. Because I regularly check my inflammatory markers, I saw that several were higher than I wanted them to be. This meant I was moving in the wrong direction on the autoimmune spectrum. I knew something was wrong, and I needed to figure out what. After lots of testing and lots of digging, my husband, Xavier, and I discovered that there was toxic mold in our house. We moved to a newly built apartment, and I became even more ill from the off-gassing of the building materials, wall-to-wall carpeting, and composite wood cabinets. I became so sensitive to certain chemicals that even just leaving the house was a risk because I never knew what would cause me to break out in a bright red rash. I became so sick that I actually slept on our outdoor balcony for a month, just so I could know that I was breathing fresh, clean air at night. Poor Xavier, who doesn't have the genes to be affected by toxic mold, stood by me as we moved from apartment to apartment for almost a year, trying to get me well. How bittersweet to spend our first wedding anniversary so unsettled and grappling with health issues!

The important lesson in this story is that life happens to *all* of us. Even the healthiest of us can move in the wrong direction on the autoimmune spectrum and experience symptoms again because of circumstances that are out of our control. That's why it's so important to remember that you always have the power to work your way back toward symptom-free optimal health by getting 100 percent back on board with The Myers Way. That's what I did, and I am back to feeling great again after detoxing from the toxic mold and following the four-pillar approach to health that I lay out in *The Autoimmune Solution*.

Now I want to share a different type of story. In the last chapter ("A World of Hope") of *The Autoimmune Solution*, I wrote about how I helped my dad reverse his autoimmunity. For those of you who haven't read it, I'll tell you a little bit about my dad. He suffered from polymyositis, an autoimmune disorder that attacks the muscles, causing extreme weakness and severe pain. Conventional medicine's approach to polymyositis is to prescribe potent medications that suppress the immune system. For him they prescribed prednisone, methotrexate, and mycophenolate mofetil (CellCept). Once my dad started taking these medications, he developed repeated infections and was constantly in and out of the hospital because his immune system was so suppressed by the very medications that were supposed to be making him well.

I persuaded Dad to take a functional medicine approach to his health and try The Myers Way by changing his diet, healing his gut, taming the toxins, healing infections, and relieving stress. Within thirty days, he was a new person! He had stopped taking all his immunosuppressive medications. He lost fifteen pounds and became more mobile. When his creatine phosphokinase (CPK) levels were checked to test for muscle damage, they were completely normal. Best of all, when my dad got the exciting news about his CPK levels, he called me and said, "Amy, you saved my life!" Can you imagine what it's like for a daughter to hear those words from her father? Even better was the fact that now that he was off those terrible medications, he didn't get sick or need to be hospitalized even once in the two years after he started The Myers Way.

Then, while I was in the middle of dealing with my own health crisis, Dad called me to say that he had a "flare" of his polymyositis and his muscle weakness and severe pain had returned. Normally, I would have jumped in immediately to uncover the root causes that led to the flare-up so that he could address them head-on using lifestyle changes. However, I was struggling to get well myself, so my dad ended up going back on the high doses of prednisone and methotrexate at the recommendation of his doctors.

Six months later, and two days after Xavier and I had moved into our new, toxin-free home, ready to start our new lives together, I received a phone call telling me that my dad was in the ICU in septic shock from pneumonia. "He's not going to make it," I was told. Our family was heartbroken, and the recent years during which my dad had been able to live symptom-free were even more precious to us, knowing now that they would be his last.

His death was all the more tragic for me because I believe that if we could have naturally addressed what had caused his flare-up, he could have avoided going back on the immune-suppressing medications and may never have developed pneumonia.

One silver lining is that I was able to share the news before my dad died that Xavier and I were going to be parents—we adopted our precious daughter Elle a few weeks after his death.

My dad's unnecessary early death and the birth of my daughter have made me more committed than ever to empowering people to take back their health and to know that autoimmunity can be prevented and reversed. I don't want what happened to me, my dad, and to so many of you and your loved ones to ever happen again. No one should have to choose between taking potentially life-threatening medications or living with debilitating symptoms. And no one should lose loved ones because of the side effects of destructive treatments offered by conventional medicine.

AUTOIMMUNITY IN AMERICA

Following are the estimated figures on the incidence of autoimmune disorders in the United States. Some of these conditions are considered autoimmune disorders and some merely resemble autoimmunity. For all these disorders and more, however, The Myers Way is an effective protocol to reverse the progression of the disease, ease its symptoms, and restore you to a healthy, vigorous life.

Graves' disease: 10 million

Psoriasis: 7.5 million

Fibromyalgia: 5 million

Lupus: 3.5 million

Celiac disease: 3 million

Hashimoto's thyroiditis: 3 million

Rheumatoid arthritis: 3 million

Chronic fatigue syndrome: 1 million

Crohn's disease: 700,000

Ulcerative colitis: 700,000

Multiple sclerosis: 250,000 to 350,000

Scleroderma: 300,000

Diabetes type 1: 25,000 to 50,000

EIGHT MAJOR MYTHS ABOUT AUTOIMMUNE CONDITIONS

Myth One: Autoimmune disorders cannot be reversed.

Myth Two: Your symptoms won't disappear without harsh medications.

Myth Three: When you treat an autoimmune disorder with medication, the side effects are no big deal.

Myth Four: Improving digestion and gut health have no effect on the progression of an autoimmune disorder.

Myth Five: Going gluten-free won't make any difference to your autoimmune disorder.

Myth Six: Having an autoimmune disorder dooms you to a poor quality of life.

Myth Seven: When it comes to autoimmune disorders, only your genes matter; environmental factors do not matter.

Myth Eight: Your immune system is what it is; there is nothing you can do to support it.

Motivated by my continued commitment to my mission, I wrote this book, *The Autoimmune Solution Cookbook,* to provide a comprehensive resource for preventing and reversing the full spectrum of inflammatory autoimmune symptoms and diseases.

Because of the enormous role that food plays in the path to healing, I know that many of you have seen amazing results from changing your diet and following The Myers Way. And the key to maintaining lifelong health is to make the healing lifestyle changes a way of life. That's why I call my program The Myers Way. I wrote this cookbook to make this way of life even easier and more convenient for you by providing delicious, healing recipes that you can make time and time again. I also wrote this book because now that you know the harm that certain foods can do to your health, food may have become something that causes you fear or anxiety. It is challenging to worry about whether any bite of food may lead to a flare-up or return of the symptoms you have worked so hard to eliminate. You no longer need to worry. Every recipe in this book will help you heal, and not only that, every recipe will be delicious. It is time to exhale with relief and love your food again.

The recipes in *The Autoimmune Solution Cookbook* are simple and use just a handful of pure, healing ingredients. The comprehensive shopping section ("Foods to Enjoy" and "Foods to Toss") makes you an informed consumer who knows exactly which healing foods and toxin-free products to purchase. You will feel a sense of power knowing that the nourishing foods you eat are helping to prevent and reverse inflammatory symptoms. Most of all, you will discover that having an autoimmune disorder doesn't need to stop you from living the life you want and that you deserve.

If you have read *The Autoimmune Solution* and already followed its thirty-day protocol, this cookbook is a perfect companion for spicing up your diet and adding more variety to your mealtimes. In it you will find a few recipes that slightly branch out from the protocol, using a few new ingredients such as maple syrup and organic coconut sugar. If you're not quite ready for these foods because you're still working to reverse your condition, you can always skip over or modify them for now and try them when your symptoms have fully resolved.

If you are new to The Myers Way, this cookbook contains a perfect introduction to my approach to preventing and reversing autoimmunity and includes everything you need to begin following the protocol. If you would like a deeper dive into The Myers Way, a six-week online program called The Myers Way Autoimmune Solution Program is available on my website (AmyMyersMD.com); in it, I walk you through the entire program step-by-step in more than six hours of videos. You can follow that program or read *The Autoimmune Solution* while enjoying the delicious recipes found here.

As a comprehensive, informative, and user-friendly resource, *The Autoimmune Solution Cookbook* includes:

- A brief look at autoimmunity, including a list of autoimmune diseases and symptoms

- Lists of foods to enjoy and foods to toss in order to prevent and reverse autoimmunity

- The Myers Way Symptom Tracker to help you understand where you fall on the autoimmune spectrum so you can determine whether you are at risk of developing an autoimmune condition, or whether you may already have one

- A review of the four pillars of The Myers Way protocol to reverse autoimmune disease:

  1. Heal Your Gut

  2. Get Rid of Gluten, Grains, and Legumes

  3. Tame the Toxins

  4. Heal Your Infections and Relieve Your Stress

- A guide for stocking your kitchen with autoimmune solution–friendly ingredients—some familiar, some that may be new to you—including fruits and vegetables, meat and seafood, and herbs and spices, as well as details on coconut products and substitutes for gluten-free and grain-free flours

- Information on buying kitchen tools and equipment—blenders, juicers, pots, and storage containers—to make your cooking easier and your life healthier

- Over 150 healing, wholesome, and innovative recipes for healthy breakfasts, on-the-go-lunches, flavorful main courses with recommended side dishes, and even decadent desserts as well as DIY home cleaners and body products that will help reverse your autoimmune symptoms and restore you to health and vitality

- Full-color photographs to show you exactly what these mouth-watering meals look like

- Informative tips and tricks to make following The Myers Way even easier, including how to stick with the program while traveling and eating out, and online resources where you can buy approved foods and ingredients without even leaving your home

With *The Autoimmune Solution*, so many of you have already reversed your autoimmune symptoms and prevented disease. And now, this cookbook will make it even easier to stay the course. It is time to enjoy delicious, nutritious, and healing foods with peace of mind. And, if you're just beginning your health journey, it's time to jumpstart your recovery! After eating the nourishing recipes in this book, your symptoms will start to improve; joint pain will lessen, skin rashes will disappear, energy and sleep will be restored—and that's just the beginning. *The Autoimmune Solution Cookbook* is your guide to preventing autoimmunity and reversing it completely.

It's time to live your very best life! Let's go!

Part One

Live the Solution

1

My Journey

When I was in my second year of medical school, I developed a long list of inexplicable symptoms: panic attacks, significant weight loss, weak legs, insomnia, anxiety, dizziness, heart palpitations, fatigue. My primary care doctor told me that I was just "stressed out" by the rigors of medical school. "No way," I said. "I spent two years in the Peace Corps. My mother died of pancreatic cancer four months after she was diagnosed. I know what stress is. There's something else going on." I insisted on a complete medical workup. The results showed that I wasn't "stressed out" or a hypochondriac or losing my mind. I had Graves' disease, an autoimmune condition in which the thyroid gland attacks itself and produces too much thyroid hormone.

My primary care doctor referred me to an endocrinologist, who offered me three choices for treatment: medication, surgical removal of my thyroid, or ablation, that is, swallowing a radioactive pill (I-131) to kill my thyroid gland. After looking high and low for natural solutions, I chose what I thought was the lesser of the three evils: taking a drug called propylthiouracil (PTU). After I had been taking it for a few weeks, my skin was dry, my hair was falling out, and I could barely get out of bed. I returned to the endocrinologist, who ran several blood tests, which revealed that I had toxic hepatitis. The PTU was destroying my liver. I needed to stop taking it immediately, get in bed until my liver recovered, and decide whether I wanted to do surgery or ablation.

Within a few days of stopping the PTU, my hyperthyroid symptoms of anxiety, insomnia, and heart palpitations became worse than before I had started the medication, yet I was still exhausted and needed my liver to recover so I could attend my medical school classes. I was scared, miserable, and felt hopeless. I was so stressed that I worried I might have to drop out of medical school. I had to choose surgery or ablation, and I went with the ablation—which remains the greatest regret of my life.

Instinctively, I knew that there had to be a better way to deal with disease and illness beyond prescribing harsh medications or killing or surgically removing vital organs. The ablation did "kill" my thyroid, and initially my symptoms worsened because large amounts of thyroid hormone were being released into my bloodstream. I experienced mood swings. I was exhausted yet I had trouble sleeping. I developed irritable bowel syndrome. I didn't want to leave my home for fear that I would have a panic attack in public. And then, all of sudden, my thyroid gland did a 180-degree turn and wasn't producing enough hormone. I gained ten pounds. My hair started falling out. I was always cold. And here's the really crazy part: my thyroid lab tests came back normal!

I was able to finish medical school and complete my residency training in emergency medicine. I became an attending emergency physician at a trauma center. As an ER doctor, I treated many people who needed immediate medical treatment as well as those who had chronic problems related to asthma and other respiratory ailments, heart and kidney disease, digestive issues, and diabetes, to name a few. It was heartbreaking to see how little conventional medicine could do to help them, other than prescribe more medications.

I worked about fifteen shifts a month, which allowed me time on my days off to study other types of medicine and more natural ways to treat chronic illness. On one of my days off, I attended a symposium on functional medicine, a relatively new field. And I found what I had been looking for. Functional medicine views the body as one unified system that deserves to be treated as such. I discovered that the type of foods we eat, leaky gut, toxins, infections, and stress are the root causes of most chronic illnesses. I also learned that the body has the ability to use its own resources to heal. Everything clicked into place. I knew this was the kind of medicine I wanted to practice. I jumped headlong into training, and before long I set up my own functional medicine practice.

What hit home personally was discovering the connection between gluten and autoimmune disease, especially thyroid conditions. I stopped eating gluten, dairy, soy, grains, and legumes; and I started to eat meat again after being a vegetarian for twenty-seven years. I healed my gut by treating infections, such as Candida overgrowth and small intestinal bacterial overgrowth (SIBO). I worked to rid my body and my environment of toxins and learned how to better handle stress. In thirty days, I was a new person. I was finally "myself" again. I had boundless energy. No intestinal problems. No anxiety. If I could reverse *my* autoimmune symptoms, surely I could help others with similar symptoms and conditions. So I developed The Myers Way, a step-by-step protocol to address the root causes of autoimmune disease.

If you have an autoimmune disease, then somewhere along the way your immune system went rogue and began attacking your own tissues. For example, if you have Hashimoto's disease, your immune system has attacked your thyroid gland. A diagnosis of rheumatoid arthritis means your immune system has gone after your joints. Multiple sclerosis indicates that your central nervous system is compromised. The list goes on and on because there are more than one hundred autoimmune diseases, and no matter which part of your body is under siege, the culprit is your immune system. This means that in order to treat, prevent, and reverse autoimmune disease, you need to get your immune system back in balance.

Conventional medicine does not recognize autoimmune diseases as diseases of the immune system. Instead, they are treated as diseases of particular organs. Unfortunately, this means that there isn't a unified branch in medicine to treat autoimmune conditions. With cancer, for example, we have specialists, oncologists, who treat many different types of cancers no matter which organ system they involve. While there are some sub-specialties within oncology, they typically still fall under one main oncology umbrella.

If, on the other hand, you are diagnosed with an autoimmune disease, you will see a specialist who focuses only on the organ system that is being affected: a rheumatologist for rheumatoid arthritis; an endocrinologist for Hashimoto's disease, Graves' disease, and diabetes; a gastroenterologist for celiac disease, ulcerative colitis, and Crohn's disease; a dermatologist for psoriasis; and so on. If you have multiple autoimmune conditions, as many people do, you will have to see several different specialists, each of whom will likely prescribe a different medication, many of which are toxic to your system and have debilitating side effects. They'll tell you that diet, lifestyle, gut health, toxins, and stress have nothing to do with your symptoms.

As a conventional physician I was trained that once you have an autoimmune condition, there's nothing you can do to reverse it. You can only manage the symptoms. That often involves taking harsh medications that suppress your entire immune system, often causing many unwanted side effects, such as fatigue, weight gain, depression, increased infection rates, and even cancer. Thankfully, there is another way.

As a functional medicine physician, I seek to find the root cause of illness, rather than just treating the symptoms with medications and invasive procedures, as conventional medicine doctors do. I describe functional medicine as "individual" medicine. You are unique. You and your body are one of a kind, not one of the ten or more separate systems—such as endocrine, respiratory, and cardiovascular—recognized by conventional medicine. I believe that head-to-toe, inside-and-out, every part of you is intimately connected to the whole of you. You deserve to be treated as an individual, not as someone with a list of textbook symptoms that could apply to anyone else.

When you visit conventional physicians, they may diagnose your fatigue, joint pain, photosensitivity, extreme sensitivity to cold in your hands and feet, recurring facial rash, and fever as lupus. They tell you to get more rest, take steroids, stay out of the sun, and wear fur-lined gloves and boots. That's not good enough for me. I don't want to treat just the symptoms. I want to know what's causing them before we take a course of action. I work with you using my four-pillar program, The Myers Way, which is described in chapter 2.

Acute inflammation is a systemic immune response that can actually help you heal. Let's say you cut your finger. You apply a bandage and go about your business. A few hours later, the wound site is red, warm to the touch, and perhaps throbbing. Your body's inflammatory response has increased the blood flow to the area as part of the healing process. Acute inflammation is a short-term, natural process. Once the situation is stabilized—your cut finger heals—your immune system has done its job. But what happens when your immune system doesn't recognize that the job is done? The system goes haywire, and uncontrolled inflammation begins to attack healthy tissue. That's called *chronic inflammation,* and it can lead to autoimmune disease. Know that not all chronic inflammation leads to autoimmune disorders; however, if you are on the autoimmune spectrum, increased inflammation can push you in the wrong direction along the spectrum and into one of more than one hundred autoimmune disorders.

Autoimmunity and Inflammatory Symptoms

Autoimmune diseases can strike any part of the body. The first step in diagnosing an autoimmune disease is to know what symptoms to look for. As you can see from this list, symptoms vary widely.

Acid reflux	Arthritis
Acne	Asthma
Attention-deficit/hyperactivity disorder (ADD/ADHD)	Blood clots
Allergies	"Brain fog"
Alzheimer's disease	Cardiovascular disease
Anxiety	Depression

Digestive issues (diarrhea, gas, bloating, indigestion, constipation, reflux/heartburn)

Dry eyes

Eczema

Fatigue

Fibrocystic breasts

Gallstones

Hair loss

Headaches

Infertility

Joint pain

Muscle pain

Obesity or excess weight gain, especially around the middle

Pancreatitis

Sleep issues (problems falling asleep and/or staying asleep)

Swollen, red, or painful joints

Uterine fibroids

Vitamin B12 deficiency

None	Some	Mild	Moderate	Severe	Diagnosis of
No inflammation	1 symptom* 1–2 times per month	1–2 symptoms* 1–2 times per week	2–3 symptoms* most days	>3 symptoms* every day	autoimmune disease

*Symptoms defined on The Myers Way Symptom Tracker

The Myers Way Symptom Tracker

Rate the following symptoms over the past seven days on a scale of 0 to 4 based on severity. 0 = None, 1 = Some, 2 = Mild, 3 = Moderate, 4 = Severe

Head

____headaches

____migraines

____faintness

____trouble sleeping

Total ____

Mind

____brain fog

____poor memory

____impaired coordination

____difficulty deciding

____slurred/stuttered speech

____learning/attention deficit

Total ____

Eyes

____swollen, red eyelids

____dark circles

____puffy eyes

____poor vision

____watery, itchy eyes

Total ____

Nose

____nasal congestion

____excessive mucus

____stuffy/runny nose

____sinus problems

____frequent sneezing

Total ____

Ears

____itchy ears

____earaches, infections

____drainage from ear

____ringing ears, hearing loss

Total ____

Mouth, Throat

____chronic cough

____frequent throat clearing

____sore throat

____swollen lips

____canker sores

Total ____

Heart

____irregular heartbeat

____rapid heartbeat

____chest pain

Total ____

Lungs

____chest congestion

____asthma, bronchitis

____shortness of breath

____difficulty breathing

Total ____

(Continued)

Skin

____acne

____hives, eczema, dry skin

____hair loss

____hot flashes

____excessive sweating

Total ____

Weight

____inability to lose weight

____food cravings

____excess weight

____insufficient weight

____compulsive eating

____water retention, swelling

Total ____

Digestion

____nausea, vomiting

____diarrhea

____constipation

____bloating

____belching, passing gas

____heartburn, indigestion

____intestinal/stomach pain or cramps

Total ____

Emotions

____anxiety

____depression

____mood swings

____nervousness

____irritability

Total ____

Energy, Activity

____fatigue

____lethargy

____hyperactivity

____restlessness

Total ____

Joints, Muscles

____joint pain/aches

____arthritis

____muscle stiffness

____muscle pain/aches

____weakness, tiredness

Total____

Other

____frequent illness/infections

____frequent/urgent urination

____genital itch, discharge

____anal itch

Total ____

Preliminary total _____

Now answer the following questions and add the points to the preliminary total to get your overall total:

1. Do you have an autoimmune disease? If yes, add 80 points. _____
2. Do you have more than one autoimmune disease? If yes, add 100 points. _____
3. Do you have elevated inflammatory markers, such as ESR (erythrocyte sedimentation rate), CRP (C-reactive protein), or homocysteine? If yes, add 10 points. _____
4. Do you have any diagnosis ending with "itis," such as arthritis, colitis, pancreatitis, sinusitis, or diverticulitis? If yes, add 10 points. _____
5. Do you have a first-degree relative (a parent or sibling) with an autoimmune disease? If yes, add 10 points for the first relative and add 2 points for each additional first-degree relative. _____
6. Do you have a second-degree relative (a grandparent, aunt, or uncle) with an autoimmune disease? If yes, add 5 points. _____
7. Are you female? If yes, add 5 points. _____

Overall total _____

Your Place on the Autoimmune Spectrum

<5	5–9	10–19	20–39	40–79	>80
No risk	Some risk	Mild risk	Moderate risk	Severe risk	

Take your overall total from The Myers Way Symptom Tracker.

If your overall total is less than 5, congratulations! Your inflammation is very low, and at this point you are unlikely to develop an autoimmune condition. For lifelong protection, follow The Myers Way to keep your inflammation at this healthy level.

If your overall total is from 5 to 9, you are at the low end of the autoimmune spectrum— but you *are* on the spectrum. You have a few risk factors for autoimmunity, raising the possibility that you might develop an autoimmune condition. To reduce your risk and lower your inflammation, follow The Myers Way.

If your overall total is from 10 to 30, you are in the middle of the autoimmune spectrum, with significant symptoms that reveal considerable inflammation and mild to moderate risk of developing autoimmunity. You can reverse your condition, heal your symptoms, and avoid the risk of an autoimmune condition by following The Myers Way.

If your overall total is over 30, you are at moderate risk either because you have one or more close family members with the condition or because you already have progressed quite far along the autoimmune spectrum. You may already have been diagnosed with an autoimmune condition, or you may have a condition that has not yet been diagnosed. If you do not currently have an autoimmune disorder, your family history and/or high levels of inflammation put you at risk for one. To reverse course and restore optimal health, follow The Myers Way.

2

The Four Pillars of The Myers Way®

Can autoimmune diseases be reversed? The answer is an unequivocal Yes! I see it time and time again with the thousands of people who come to my clinic. Identifying the root causes of your autoimmune disease is the first step in reversing your symptoms and healing your body. I designed the four pillars of The Myers Way to address the root causes of autoimmune disease that I have identified during my decade of clinical experience working with thousands of autoimmune patients. Here's a brief summary of how The Myers Way works and its four pillars. If you have read my previous books, use this chapter as a refresher. If you're living with or cooking for someone who has an autoimmune disease, this chapter will help you understand why your loved one follows The Myers Way and how powerful it is.

1. Heal Your Gut

The intestinal tract, or the gut, starts at the mouth and ends at the anus. I always say that the gut is the "gateway to health" since nearly 80 percent of your immune system is located there. If your gut isn't healthy, then your immune system isn't healthy either. However, we know from physician and researcher Dr. Alessio Fasano that a condition known as *leaky gut* is a necessary precursor for autoimmunity, meaning that if you have an auto-immune disease, at some point you developed leaky gut.

Leaky gut happens when the tight junctions that hold your intestinal wall together become loose. Think of your gut lining as a drawbridge. Teeny tiny boats (macronutrients and micronutrients in food) that are meant to get through the bridge do so without a problem. This is how vital nutrients from the food you eat get absorbed into your bloodstream. However, certain lifestyle and environmental factors will cause that drawbridge to open, allowing bigger boats to cross into the bloodstream that aren't meant to. When that happens, your gut is considered to be "leaky," and microbes, toxins, proteins, and partially digested food particles that were never meant to pass through the drawbridge are able to get into your bloodstream.

The top causes of leaky gut are:

- Toxic and inflammatory foods, particularly gluten because it triggers the release of the protein zonulin, which signals the tight junctions of your intestinal wall to open up and stay open

- Gut infections such as Candida overgrowth, SIBO, and parasites

- Some medications, including antibiotics; nonsteroidal anti-inflammatory drugs (NSAIDs), such as Motrin and Advil; steroids; birth control pills and other hormones; and antacids

- Chronic stress

Once your gut is leaky and food particles such as gluten and dairy, microbes, viruses, and toxins are flooding your bloodstream, your immune system marks these escaped substances as dangerous invaders and creates inflammation to get rid of them. As your gut remains leaky and more and more particles escape into your bloodstream, your immune system sends out wave after wave of inflammation. Eventually, it becomes overstressed and begins firing less accurately. This leads to autoimmunity as your own tissues end up in the crosshairs of your overworked immune system.

On top of this, your immune system starts making antibodies against the specific escaped substances in your bloodstream because it recognizes them as foreign invaders. Many of these foreign invaders look very similar to your own body's cells. Your immune system can get confused and accidentally attack your tissues in a process of mistaken identity called *molecular mimicry*. Gluten and dairy are common culprits behind molecular mimicry, particularly in autoimmune thyroid conditions (Hashimoto's and Graves' diseases).

The good news is that by repairing your gut, you can put an end to the inflammation and molecular mimicry that are causing your autoimmune symptoms and can stop your body from attacking itself. To do this, I recommend a "4R" approach to repairing your gut.

1. **REMOVE** the bad. The goal is to get rid of anything that negatively affects the environment of your gastrointestinal tract, such as toxic and inflammatory foods (see page 77) and gastric irritants such as alcohol, caffeine, or medications. Luckily, you are on the right track with this cookbook because every recipe included here is free of any of the toxic and inflammatory foods that cause your gut to become leaky. In addition, it is critical to get rid of any gut infections such as Candida overgrowth, SIBO, or parasites. (I have a free symptoms quiz on my website to help you determine whether you have Candida overgrowth, SIBO, or parasites. You can find it at amymd.io/quiz.)

   If you do have Candida overgrowth or SIBO, I recommend minimizing your intake of carbohydrates (such as baked goods, waffles, and pancakes) and starchy vegetables (such as sweet potatoes and squash) and eating no more than 2 cups per day of fruit until these gut infections have resolved. Additionally, I recommend

---

How to Know if You Have Candida Overgrowth, SIBO, or Parasites and What to Do About It, visit amymd.io/quiz.

---

following my supplement protocols for beating these infections, which you can find at amymd.io/gutinfections.

2. **RESTORE** the good. In this step you add back in the essential ingredients for proper digestion and absorption that may have been depleted by diet, medications (such as antacids) disease, or aging. Adding back digestive enzymes in supplement form is one key component of this step (see chapter 18 for more information on the supplements I recommend). Without these enzymes, you don't digest food properly, which stresses your digestive system and reduces your ability to fully absorb the healing nutrients in your food. Some people also need to restore their stomach acid with supplemental hydrochloric acid (HCl) if they are dealing with heartburn or acid reflux.

3. **REINOCULATE** with healthy bacteria. Restoring beneficial bacteria to reestablish a healthy balance of good bacteria is critical. This can be accomplished by taking a high-quality, high-concentration probiotic supplement that contains beneficial bacteria such as *Bifidobacterium* and *Lactobacillus*. I start my patients with leaky gut on a daily dose of 100 billion CFUs (colony-forming units), and I recommend 30 billion CFUs daily for gut health maintenance.

4. **REPAIR** the gut. Providing the nutrients necessary to help the gut repair itself is essential. One of my favorite supplements is The Myers Way Collagen Protein®, which is rich in amino acids that "seal the leaks" or perforations in your gut by healing damaged cells and building new tissue. I believe collagen is so vital to healing a leaky gut that I use it throughout this cookbook. Another one of my favorite supplements is L-glutamine, an amino acid that helps your gut cells turn over faster so that your gut lining can repair itself.

Eating the right foods and taking gut-repairing supplements are the first steps to healing your gut and reversing the symptoms of autoimmunity. The recipes in *The Autoimmune Solution Cookbook* help you stay the course for smooth sailing with recipes for gut-healing smoothies, bone broths, teas, soups, and more. As you enjoy the recipes in this book, you'll know that your gut is healed when your digestive issues and food sensitivities disappear, your skin issues clear up, your autoimmune lab results improve, and you return to your optimal self.

2. Get Rid of Gluten, Grains, and Legumes

"Gluten-free? That's just some crazy fad people are trying to cash in on. We've been eating wheat for thousands of years, so why all of a sudden would it turn out not to be healthy?"

That's what many people believe about the role of gluten in our health, and most conventional doctors are no different. Tell your doctor that you are concerned about gluten, and he or she will most likely say two things: "We can run a blood test and see whether you have celiac disease," and "Do you have any digestive issues? No? Then you don't have to worry about gluten."

This couldn't be farther from the truth. Gluten sensitivity, or non-celiac gluten sensitivity (the scientifically agreed-upon term), can cause a whole host of symptoms beyond digestive issues, including fatigue, brain fog, hormonal imbalances, skin issues, inflammation, depression, anxiety, and more. And, while celiac disease is in fact rare, gluten sensitivity is quite common, although most people don't know they have it. An estimated 99 percent of people with celiac disease or gluten sensitivity are undiagnosed.

So how does gluten affect autoimmunity? Remember, gluten is the most common cause of leaky gut because of the zonulin your body releases every time you eat it. It also increases your overall inflammation if you have gluten sensitivity, causing your immune system to go haywire. Furthermore, as I mentioned earlier, gluten can actually cause your immune system to attack your own tissues by mistake because of molecular mimicry.

I want to point out that our modern-day gluten is not the same gluten that your grandparents ate. Today's wheat has been hybridized to be resistant to insects and drought and to grow faster than older strains of wheat. The result is a harder-to-digest, inflammation-causing grain that contains much more gluten than its predecessor. Second, modern gluten is *deamidated,* which means it can be dissolved in water, and because of that it has been added to an enormous range of foods and products that it was never meant to be in. These two factors mean that we are not only eating a different kind of gluten than our ancestors ate, we are eating and being exposed to much more of it.

If you have autoimmunity, the most important thing to take away from this book is to *stop eating gluten now and forever.* The "forever" part is key because research has shown that eating gluten can elevate your gluten antibodies for up to three months, meaning that even if you eat gluten only four times a year, you will be in a state of inflammation year-round.

It's easy to avoid gluten when the enemy is hiding in plain sight such as in pastas, breads, baked goods, snack foods, and cereals. What most people don't know is that gluten can be lurking in hundreds of thousands of foods, often in the least expected ones, such as chicken stock, soy sauce, ketchup, mustard, barbecue sauce, chewing gum, and blended coffees. That's why I recommend making your own stocks, sauces, and condiments when possible using recipes such as those in chapter 9. If you do need to purchase store-bought pantry items, check out chapter 3 and Resources for recommended brands and stores for gluten-free versions of these products.

Gluten can even be lurking in your lipstick, lotion, and shampoo, so I have included recipes for homemade body products in chapter 12 as well as my favorite online places to shop for makeup and body products (see Resources).

In addition to ditching gluten, I also recommend that all of my autoimmune patients eliminate grains and legumes for the first thirty days of The Myers Way. This sometimes comes as a shock to people, particularly vegetarians who think of these food groups as staples of a healthy diet. I myself was a vegetarian for twenty-seven years! However, grains and legumes contain a problematic group of substances called *lectins.* Lectins are proteins that help keep two carbohydrate molecules together. They are found in animals, plants, and microorganisms, and the ones to be concerned about are those in grains, where they are plentiful, and legumes, where they are less plentiful yet still concerning.

One problematic type of lectin that is especially bad for people with celiac disease is called *prolamin*, which is found in quinoa, corn, and oats. Although in theory, people with celiac disease can eat nongluten and pseudograins such as quinoa, in reality the prolamins in these supposedly safe foods damage their guts and stimulate their immune systems. Prolamins can also have that effect on those of us who have other types of autoimmune conditions or who are somewhere on the autoimmune spectrum. This is because prolamin interacts poorly with your brush border—the all-important portion of your small intestine full of villi and microvilli. You want to protect, rather than stress, those delicate parts of your digestive tract.

In addition, prolamins behave much like the proteins in gluten. And if you have an autoimmune or inflammatory condition, your immune system is already compromised in the presence of gluten. An overstressed immune system cannot tell the difference between gluten and its look-alikes, so you'll want to avoid both of them.

Grains and legumes also contain *agglutinins*, which have been shown to cause leaky gut and disrupt your immune system by stimulating the immune system and binding with immune cells.

For these reasons, the second pillar of The Myers Way is eliminating gluten, grains, and legumes from your diet for at least thirty days. During these thirty days, I also recommend avoiding dairy, eggs, nightshade vegetables, and toxic foods such as sugar, caffeine, alcohol, and genetically modified organisms (GMOs), which also contribute to leaky gut. After thirty days, you may slowly reintroduce some of these foods into your diet (I walk you through how to do that in chapter 17). If the inflammatory symptoms return, then you know to eliminate those particular foods entirely from your diet (I call these your *"absolute no"* foods), and if you don't experience symptoms, then you'll know that you can tolerate them in moderation or on special occasions.

Best of all, you can rest easy knowing that every recipe in *The Autoimmune Solution Cookbook* is free from all toxic and inflammatory foods and is designed to help you move toward the optimal health side of the autoimmune spectrum and stay there.

3. Tame the Toxins

Toxins are substances that are dangerous to the human body. These include heavy metals such as lead, mercury, and cadmium; industrial chemicals, pollutants, pesticides, molds, and the volatile organic compounds they release; and countless other chemicals.

Unfortunately, toxins can be found all around us. They are in the air we breathe, the water we drink, the foods we eat, and the products we use in our homes and on our bodies. More than eighty thousand chemicals currently are used in the United States, and most of them have not been properly tested for their health effects. On top of that, most products don't contain just one chemical, and if a product is made up of five ingredients, for instance, regulatory agencies test each one *separately* for safety—not all five together. Take a look at any of the cleaning solutions under your sink or the beauty products in your bathroom and you'll see that the number of potentially dangerous chemicals you're exposed to daily is staggering. And that doesn't even account for all of the toxic herbicides, pesticides, and GMOs that can be found in conventionally farmed foods.

The effects of all these toxins on our bodies are complex. After all, thousands of industrial chemicals are out there, and we're just beginning to understand how they work on the body—not to mention how they work in conjunction with one another. What we do know is that a heavy toxic burden puts you at greater risk for developing an autoimmune disease, and there are a few theories as to why.

One thought is that certain toxins, especially heavy metals, physically damage your tissues. Your immune system no longer recognizes these damaged cells as part of your own body and attacks them, thinking they're foreign invaders. Another theory is that the damage inflicted by toxins elicits an inflammatory response from the immune system. The constant assault of chronic exposure puts the immune system on high alert, and it begins attacking everything—including your own tissues.

I'm sharing all of this with you not to frighten you or stress you out. My goal is to empower you to recognize the health effects that these toxins are having on you so that you can make smart choices to tame your toxic burden. I like to break these choices into two main toxin-taming strategies: *prevention* and *detoxification*.

The goal of *prevention* is to minimize your exposure to toxins from the four most common ways they get into your body: through the air, the water, the foods you eat, and the home and body products you use. To do this I recommend using a HEPA filter to filter the air in your home and workspace; filtering the water you use for drinking, showering, and cooking; buying 100 percent organic, non-GMO foods; and either finding toxin-free versions of your home and body products or making your own all-natural versions (see chapter 12 and Resources).

The goal of *detoxification* is to support your body's natural ability to detoxify so that you're safely and effectively flushing toxins out of your system. My mantra for detoxing is to pee, poop, and sweat toxins out. Drink plenty of water to ensure that you're peeing and pooping, and use an infrared sauna (see Resources) or exercise lightly so that you're sweating.

Also, most of your detoxification is done through the liver, so you'll want to support your liver during this process. The nutrients you'll be eating while following The Myers Way help your liver mobilize the toxins that are in your tissues. Your body's biggest detoxifier is glutathione, so I also recommend supplementing with extra glutathione (see chapter 18 for more information on supplements) while your body is trying to excrete toxins, especially if you are anywhere on the autoimmune spectrum.

Armed with this information, you can make smart choices that will dramatically reduce your toxic burden and prevent dangerous industrial chemicals from wrecking your health. Remember, knowledge is power!

4. Heal Your Infections and Relieve Your Stress

The fourth pillar of The Myers Way is addressing the viral and bacterial infections (some of which you may have had for decades without ever knowing you had it) that can trigger autoimmunity, and managing the stress that can exacerbate these infections and wreak havoc on your immune system.

Heal Infections

No one knows exactly how infections trigger autoimmune diseases. Because our immune systems are so complicated and each infection is unique, it's likely that multiple factors are involved. Recent research has identified three leading theories that, when combined, explain the various links between infections and autoimmune disease.

Molecular Mimicry. I've already mentioned how molecular mimicry can happen with gluten, and the same principle applies to infections. If a virus or bacteria is similar enough to a type of your body's tissues, your immune system can attack your tissues by mistake.

Bystander Activation. In this situation, a bacteria or virus invades your tissues, your immune system kicks in to kill the infection, and it accidentally attacks the surrounding tissues (the "innocent bystander" in this scenario).

Cryptic Antigens. Never mind the scientific terminology here; just think of this as the "hijacking theory," because an infection (usually a virus) hijacks your cells' DNA to hide from your immune system. Your immune system is smart enough to detect the virus anyway and attacks the virus and the cells it's hiding in.

You may be thinking that this isn't something you have to worry about because you don't have any infections. Remember, I just said that you may have had an infection years ago without ever knowing it. That's because

BACTERIAL INFECTIONS AND AUTOIMMUNITY

Here's a list of the most common associations between bacterial infections and autoimmune conditions:

Type of Microbe	Associated Disorder
Campylobacter	Guillain–Barré syndrome
Chlamydia pneumoniae[1]	Multiple sclerosis
Citrobacter, Klebsiella, Proteus, Porphyromonas	Rheumatoid arthritis
E. coli, Proteus	Autoimmunity in general
Klebsiella	Ankylosing spondylitis
Streptococcus pyogenes	Rheumatic fever
Yersinia	Graves' disease, Hashimoto's thyroiditis

1. This is *not* the same bacterium that causes the sexually transmitted disease, though obviously it is from the same family.

the infection with the bacteria or virus didn't immediately present symptoms, however it has remained latent (or inactive) for years.

For example, even if you weren't teased in school for coming down with "the kissing disease" (mononucleosis), you were very likely infected with the Epstein-Barr virus (which causes mono), since 95 percent of US adults have picked it up by age forty, and it can be present without any symptoms. Once you've been infected with this virus, it never fully leaves your body, even long after symptoms have disappeared.

Research has shown a strong correlation between Epstein-Barr and numerous autoimmune diseases, including multiple sclerosis (MS), lupus, chronic fatigue syndrome, fibromyalgia, and Hashimoto's and Graves' diseases. In fact, while 95 percent of people in the US have Epstein-Barr antibodies, 100 percent of people with MS have them, meaning people who have never been exposed to Epstein-Barr don't seem to develop MS. We also know that high levels of Epstein-Barr antibodies (meaning the virus has reactivated and your immune system is mounting a response to it) are a predictor of MS symptoms and flares, and a history of infectious mono doubles your risk for developing MS.

Several bacterial infections are also associated with autoimmunity. *Yersinia* is associated with autoimmune thyroid conditions, and *Klebsiella* infections have been implicated in rheumatoid arthritis. *Campylobacter*, a ferocious bacterium, is associated with Guillain-Barré syndrome. The list goes on and on.

The best way to heal these infections and prevent them from flaring up and leading to autoimmune symptoms is to support your immune system by following all four pillars of The Myers Way. When your immune system has the support it needs and isn't constantly on high alert, it can effectively defend against a reactivation of latent infections.

Relieve Stress

You might ask, "What does stress have to do with my health?" Plenty!

As odd as it may seem, your body can be stressed by both good news (getting hired for a new job) and bad news (getting fired). In both cases, your system responds the same way.

Stress can be emotional, mental, or physical; it can come from physical injury, not getting enough sleep, exposure to toxins, ignoring a leaky gut, or even eating a diet full of inflammatory foods. Whether you're planning a wedding or struggling through a divorce, bringing a new baby into the family or losing a loved one, your body releases a torrent of stress hormones to help you cope—and chief among them is *cortisol*.

You can think of cortisol as a chemical messenger. When you're in a stressful situation, cortisol tells your immune system to gear up for a challenge. Your immune system responds by producing inflammation, and then cortisol signals your immune system to calm down when the danger has passed.

This system works well when you encounter acute stress that happens suddenly and then passes. However, when you have constant stressors—such as sleep deprivation, poor diet, long hours at work, problems with relationships—your immune system never gets to turn off. Your inflammatory immune response is activated for too long and eventually goes rogue, attacking your own body tissues. Soon, your stress hormones try to suppress the response and go overboard, leaving you with a weakened immune system. Simultaneously, your body is inflamed and you are vulnerable to infections, including latent infections such as the Epstein-Barr virus. Each time these viruses are activated, they replicate and damage more of your cells. This begins a vicious cycle: the infection becomes active and destroys tissue, provoking an even greater immune response; then your body releases cortisol to calm it down, which triggers more infection—and so on.

There are hundreds of ways to relieve stress—breathing deeply, meditating, yoga, taking a walk, playing with a pet or child, golfing, to name a few. It's important to figure out what works for *you* and what you will be able to incorporate into your daily routine so that managing your stress becomes a way of life. (See the Resources for more stress-relieving ideas.)

And let's face it, food shopping and cooking can sometimes be time-consuming and stressful in and of themselves. With *The Autoimmune Solution Cookbook*, I've taken the guesswork out of preparing and eating nourishing meals that support your health. My goal is to make it easy and completely stress-free for you to make delicious and immune-supporting meals. Tens of thousands of people have already experienced transformative healing using The Myers Way, and now, with *The Autoimmune Solution Cookbook* in your hands, it's easier than ever before.

Turn the page and let's get started!

Part Two

Ingredients and Kitchen Tools

3

What You Need
in Your Kitchen

So many people around the world (myself included) are living proof that following The Myers Way as a way of life is possible, and I'm thrilled that *The Autoimmune Solution* helped make that easier for them. However, it's not just information that makes lifestyle changes easier. Thanks to a wave of people looking to reverse their autoimmunity, approved foods and ingredients are now readily available at affordable prices in most stores and online as companies race to cater to those of us who have adopted this way of life (see Resources). Gone are the days of having to shop only at specialty grocery stores or farmers' markets (although I still highly recommend supporting your local farmers' market!).

In this chapter I list and explain ingredients that I stock in my pantry and those that you'll need for the delicious recipes in this book. You'll find detailed information on gluten-free and grain-free flours, proteins, fruits, vegetables, herbs, and spices that you'll use to make these easy and flavorful recipes. If you come across an ingredient that's new to you, just turn to this chapter for an explanation of what it is, why it is beneficial for your health, and where to purchase it.

For quick reference, this chapter also includes staple recipes I use frequently throughout this book—Cauliflower Rice (page 67), Coconut Milk (page 68), Coconut Butter (page 69), Coconut Milk Yogurt (page 70), and Gut-Healing Bone Broth (page 71)—as well as how to deal with the important staples of onions and garlic.

Note that even if it's not specifically stated in a recipe, they all call for using organic fruits, vegetables, herbs, and spices as well as grass-fed, pasture-raised meats and wild-caught seafood. The goal is to fuel your body with nourishing foods that heal, and foods that are conventionally farmed, laden with pesticides, or contain GMOs (that is, living organisms that have been altered in high-tech genetic engineering labs) are far from that! For instance, today's conventional farming practices are built around the use of GMOs, and when planted or fed to livestock, these GMOs impart toxic chemicals that are harmful to human health. What's more, foods that contain GMOs are often specifically engineered to withstand higher levels of pesticides, so they contain significantly more pesticides than non-GMO foods.

When shopping for organic items, you'll notice that there are four different types of organic label, and each has a very different meaning:

- Labels that say "100 percent organic": As the label implies, these products are made with entirely organic ingredients.

- Labels that say "USDA organic": These foods contain at least 95 percent organic ingredients.

- Labels that say "Made with organic": These foods are made with at least 70 percent organic ingredients.

- Labels that list specific organic ingredients: Companies do this when they use some organic ingredients but not enough for any of the higher certifications.

You'll want to stick with "100 percent organic" as much as possible. Here are three reasons why:

1. **Pesticides have been directly linked to autoimmune disease.**

   In one 2007 study, three hundred thousand death certificates over fourteen years showed that farmers who were exposed to pesticides while working with crops were more likely to die from a systemic autoimmune disease. Research has even linked household pesticides with an increased risk for developing autoimmune diseases, including rheumatoid arthritis and lupus.

   Many of the pesticides used in conventional farming are systemic, meaning they become an integral part of the plant and its products and cannot be washed off. An apple that has been grown in a pesticide-filled orchard, for example, has integrated the pesticides into that sweet white part that tastes so good, so washing the apple doesn't get rid of the pesticides.

2. **Non-organic meat contains growth hormones and antibiotics.**

   Conventionally raised livestock is regularly injected with engineered growth hormones that are designed to increase animal size faster so they can be slaughtered faster (for beef breeds). For dairy breeds, these growth hormones ramp up milk production to an unnatural pace. Growth hormones may also increase an insulin-like growth factor that can cause an increased risk of breast, prostate, and other cancers in humans.

   Cows, chickens, and pigs that are penned in crowded, dirty conditions are susceptible to infections and are given antibiotics to prevent disease outbreaks. The frequent use of antibiotics in livestock helps breed antibiotic-resistant "supergerms" that our immune systems have a difficult time fighting. These superbugs can be particularly dangerous in those people who are immunosuppressed, as many who take medications for autoimmune disease are.

3. **Organic produce is more nutritious.**

   A recent study showed that organic produce is richer in nutrients and antioxidants and lower in heavy metals, especially cadmium, and pesticides. Other studies suggest that good soil nutrition increases the production of cancer-fighting compounds, called *flavonoids*, and that conventional farming practices that use lots of pesticides and herbicides disturb their production.

Remember, Tame the Toxins is the third pillar of The Myers Way, and step one is *prevention*. Eating organic, grass-fed, pasture-raised, and wild-caught foods will significantly reduce your exposure to toxins and decrease your overall toxic burden.

I'm often asked whether switching to all organic foods is expensive. Although it's true that purchasing organic foods can cost more, your body's health and living your life on your own terms are worth it. Plus, when you're following The Myers Way, you won't be spending money on processed foods, dairy products, and other inflammatory items, so you'll probably save money in the long run.

At the same time, organic foods and ingredients are now more affordable than ever, since more stores are carrying them. When I wrote *The Autoimmune Solution*, I shopped exclusively at my local farmers' market and Whole Foods Market. Today, the demand for organic foods has skyrocketed, so the supply and distribution of such foods have dramatically improved. I can now purchase the bulk of my organic foods at Costco and Target. We are fortunate to have a secondary freezer in our garage that allows us to purchase beef, pork, poultry, and seafood in bulk from several online retailers that I trust. We buy our grass-fed, pasture-raised meats from ButcherBox.com (see Resources) and our seafood from Vitalchoice.com (see Resources). They automatically deliver to our door each month so I don't even have to make a trip to the store!

WHEN SHOPPING FOR AND PREPARING MEALS, REMEMBER TO . . .

- **Put organic, 100 percent grass-fed, pasture-raised beef, pork, chicken, turkey, and lamb at the top of the list.** Animals are at the top of the food chain, so if they're eating GMO- and pesticide-laden feed, then you're getting those chemicals magnified many times when you eat those animals. I explain this further below under "Meat and Poultry."

- **Avoid buying the "Dirty Dozen" fruits and vegetables.** Each year the Environmental Working Group analyzes and lists in numerical order the pesticide content of approximately fifty fruits and vegetables. The "Dirty Dozen" list contains the twelve foods that have the highest concentration of pesticides, and it is a great tool for prioritizing which organic foods to purchase if you can choose organic for only some items because of budgetary concerns. Start at the top of the list and buy organic options for the first five, ten, or all twelve—whatever your budget allows. Or select the items from the list that you eat most frequently and switch to organic for those. Visit www.ewg.org to get the latest "Dirty Dozen" fruits and vegetables.

- **Eventually adopt the "Clean Fifteen."** This list, also from the Environmental Working Group, contains conventionally grown fruits and vegetables with the lowest concentration of chemicals. Buying organic for these items can be prioritized third, after meats and the "Dirty Dozen."

- **Buy in bulk.** Buying food in bulk quantities can be economical, time-saving, and environmentally sound. It makes sense to buy large quantities of coconut oil, big bunches of dark greens, and large packages of organic boneless, skinless chicken breasts because you'll cook and eat them frequently with *The Autoimmune Solution Cookbook* recipes. You will also save valuable time by shopping less frequently. When possible, use your own canvas totes and glass containers to cut down on toxic packaging and environmental waste. Pack your fruits, vegetables, and herbs in reusable shopping bags. When you get home, clean the greens and herbs before refrigerating them. Divide chicken breasts into individual portions and freeze.

- **Batch cook your meals.** Many of the recipes in *The Autoimmune Solution Cookbook* lend themselves to batch cooking, that is, preparing multiple portions of a meal and storing them to enjoy later in the week or month. Batch cooking is economical because there's less waste; it saves time; and it is less stressful, because knowing that you have cooked food or meals on hand takes the pressure off of worrying about what's for dinner. (Remember, Relieve Your Stress is part of the fourth pillar of The Myers Way!) For instance, if you stock your freezer with 1-cup portions of Gut-Healing Bone Broth (page 71) and individual servings of Cauliflower Rice (page 67) and your refrigerator is full of chopped vegetables and salad greens, you are more likely to stay on the program.

Ingredients by the Alphabet

Baking Powder

Baking powder helps baked goods rise and become fluffy. Once combined with a liquid, baking powder releases gas bubbles and the magic begins. Purchase aluminum-free baking soda, such as Rumford or Bob's Red Mill brands. (Aluminum can accumulate in the body, especially the bones.) It's easy to make your own baking powder by whisking together ¼ cup cream of tartar and 2 tablespoons baking soda. Store it in a glass jar and stir well before using to remove any clumps.

Cacao and Cocoa

Cacao Nibs and Cacao Powder Cacao is raw chocolate that hasn't been heated, treated, processed, or sweetened. Nibs are the pebblelike broken bits of cacao tree seeds. Bursting with antioxidants, essential fatty acids, and other nutrients such as magnesium and iron, cacao nibs can be added to trail mix, smoothies, and desserts. Store them in the refrigerator or at room temperature. Cacao is also available as a powder, which should be kept at room temperature.

Cocoa Powder You can use cocoa powder and cacao powder interchangeably in smoothies or when baking. If you want more nutrients, I suggest cacao powder. If you want fewer calories and a good source of antioxidants, then definitely go with cocoa powder. Avoid sugar-laden, processed hot cocoa mixes.

Coconut

What would we do without coconuts? From the white meat to the translucent water inside, organic coconut products are anti-inflammatory, metabolism boosting, and hormone balancing. Here's a guide to the various coconut foods used in *The Autoimmune Solution Cookbook*.

Coconut Aminos This liquid condiment is a great substitute for those of us who can't eat soy sauce. I love Asian food and hated giving it up as I said good-bye to soy products. When coconut aminos came onto the market, I was thrilled because it's the closest thing I have found to real soy sauce. Coconut aminos are made by aging organic coconut sap and blending it with sun-dried, mineral-rich sea salt. Use it in stir-fried dishes, dips, and dressings. Be careful not to confuse gluten-free, soy-free coconut aminos with liquid aminos, which are made from soybeans.

Coconut Butter For this butter, coconut flesh is ground into a paste, much like nut butters. Rich in healthy fat, fiber, and nutrients, coconut butter can be creamy when warmed or hard when cold. It has become readily available at most grocery stores. When added to smoothies it provides creaminess and fats to keep you feeling full for hours. If you use as much coconut butter as I do, it's easy to make your own (page 69). Be sure to try some of the flavored variations.

Coconut Flakes Coconut flakes make great additions to trail mix, granola bars, cereals, and baked goods. If you buy them, be sure to buy unsweetened flakes or shredded coconut with no added sweeteners.

Coconut Flour See under "Flours" (page 50).

Coconut Oil Coconut oil is a versatile go-to anti-inflammatory cooking fat. It has a medium to high smoke point (refer to "Smoke Points of Fats and Oils" on page 49). Add 1 or 2 tablespoons to smoothies. Use it to grease baking pans or muffin tins. Coconut oil is also a great skin and nail moisturizer. I leave my coconut oil in the cabinet to the right of my stove, however you can also refrigerate it. If chilled, bring it to room temperature for easier scooping and use.

Coconut Milk I have included a recipe to make your own Coconut Milk (page 68). If you choose to purchase it, I recommend buying 100 percent organic full-fat coconut milk that is made from coconut meat and water. Be sure to check the label; if the ingredients include anything other than coconut and water, put it back on the shelf. When I'm in a hurry and don't have time to make my own, I typically buy coconut milk in a BPA-free can.

Coconut Milk Yogurt I grew up making yogurt on Sundays with my mom, and this is a tradition I have continued with my daughter. Although Elle is a little too young to actually help me make the yogurt, she loves the finished product! In fact, when I am having a hard time getting her to eat something, I simply add a spoonful of plain coconut yogurt to her food and she gobbles it right up. I have included a recipe on page 70. Most commercial yogurts, including coconut yogurts, have added sugars, carrageenan (an inflammatory food additive), and other unwanted ingredients.

Coconut Cream You can buy this in a 15-ounce container or use the cream layer from full-fat canned coconut milk. We often have a can or two of full-fat coconut milk stored in the refrigerator so that it's only minutes from having a sweet craving to enjoying a decadent dessert. You can use the leftover milk for one of the dreamy smoothies in this cookbook.

Coconut Sugar See "Sweeteners" (page 64).

Fats

Quality fats are essential to building healthy cell membranes and helping the nervous system send messages to the brain. The right kinds of fats assist your gut in absorbing certain fat-soluble vitamins such as vitamins A, D, K, and E, which are critical to optimal immune function. And let's face it: fat makes food taste great and keeps you full longer. Removing bad industrial seed oils (canola, soy, and corn oils) and *trans* fats from your diet and replacing them with good fats (avocado, coconut, olive, and certain animal fats) is an essential step for living The Myers Way.

Keep your kitchen stocked with organic avocado, coconut, and olive oil for sautéing, cooking, and drizzling on vegetables and salads. Use bacon fat from pastured and nitrate-free bacon to cook brussels sprouts and wilt dark, leafy greens.

When it comes to those plastic bottles of so-called vegetable oils on supermarket shelves, know that the contents bear no resemblance to the plant they came from and are often grown from genetically modified seeds. The seeds of canola (rapeseed), soy, corn, sunflower, and others (not necessarily vegetables) are mechanically separated from the plants. Then they are crushed and processed with solvents, and the resulting oil is treated with more chemicals to make it look good and smell okay. These oils are a major contributor to inflammation, so avoid them at all costs.

The *smoke point* of an oil or fat (see the chart on page 49) refers to the temperature at which the oil produces a steady stream of smoke when heated. Vegetable oils have high smoke points, however, they break down when heated and release inflammatory toxins that are damaging to your system. I could go on and on, but you get the picture.

Unless otherwise noted, store oils in a cool, dark place where the temperature is constant. Extreme heat, cold, and light will affect the oil's flavor, so never refrigerate oils or keep them right next to the oven or stove. Store olive oil away from windows, even if it comes in a dark bottle. Use it within a year of purchase. The toxic chemicals in plastics get absorbed more readily into fats and oils, so when possible, purchase fats and oils in glass bottles and jars.

When it comes to cooking, it's important to choose from the healthy, healing fats and oils listed below and to know their smoke points. Avoid nut oils (walnut, hazelnut, almond, macadamia), seed oils (hemp, flax, sunflower), vegetables oils (soy, canola, safflower, corn), and peanut oil.

Avocado Oil Avocados are not just for guacamole! Avocado oil is becoming more popular because of its protective carotenoids and ability to relieve psoriasis and symptoms of arthritis, and because it is loaded with vitamin E. And those are just some of its many benefits.

Avocado oil has a high smoke point, is a monounsaturated fat, and has so many health benefits, I use it in many recipes throughout this book. It has a mild, slightly nutty flavor, yet it doesn't taste like avocados, so it's perfect for dressings and salads. Organic avocado oil is available in supermarkets and online.

And that's not all. Avocado oil can be used as a moisturizer (rub it on your dry feet and elbows), eye makeup remover, and hair conditioner.

Coconut Oil See page 46.

Olive Oil People who live in countries on the Mediterranean Sea have longer life expectancies and lower risks of developing heart disease, high blood pressure, and stroke compared with North Americans and Northern Europeans. Their consumption of lots of olive oil is known to be one contributing factor. Olive oil, a monounsaturated fat, has powerful anti-inflammatory and antibacterial properties and is ideal for supporting gut health.

SMOKE POINTS OF FATS AND OILS

Fat/Oil	Smoke Point (°F)	Smoke Point (°C)
Avocado Oil	520	271
Beef Tallow	400	205
Coconut Oil (extra virgin)	350	175
Extra Virgin Olive Oil	375	190
Flaxseed Oil	225	107
Ghee	480	250
Grapeseed Oil	420	216
Lard	370	185
Palm Oil	450	230
Toasted Sesame Oil	350	175

Let me explain what to look for when shopping for olive oil. To be labeled "organic extra virgin olive oil," the oil must contain less than 0.1 percent oleic acid. Some industrial producers use poor quality olives and a chemical process that washes away and reduces the extra acid so it can still be labeled "extra virgin." Other producers mix lesser grade oils from various countries. The label on a quality extra virgin olive oil will note where the olives were grown and pressed. Use your best extra virgin olive oil for drizzling on fish, salads, and vegetables. Avoid anything labeled "light olive oil" because it's mixed with refined or lesser quality oils. Your health and your immune system will thank you for splurging on the organic extra virgin olive oil in a dark glass bottle.

Palm Shortening This is another ingredient that has become mainstream since I wrote *The Autoimmune Solution*, and it has transformed the ability to make and eat delicious autoimmune-friendly baked goods such as crackers, muffins, cookies, and cakes. Palm shortening is a combination of palm tree oil (not from a coconut palm tree) and coconut oil. It is ideal for baking because it is shelf stable and neutral in flavor, and it has a firm texture, a high smoke point, and no *trans* fats. I use it throughout this cookbook.

Toasted Sesame Oil Sesame oil is a good source of vitamin E, magnesium, zinc, calcium, copper, and iron—all powerful autoimmunity fighters. Toasted sesame oil imparts a mild, nutty flavor to marinades, stir-fried dishes, and other Asian dishes. It is made by toasting sesame seeds before they are pressed; the resulting oil is golden brown in color. I recommend buying cold-pressed, organic, golden brown toasted sesame seed oil, not the yellowish ones in a glass bottle. Please note, sesame oil has a very low smoke point. Once opened, store it in the refrigerator.

Fish Sauce

A condiment used in Southeast Asian cooking, fish sauce is made from fermented fish and salt. A little bit goes a long way, so use it sparingly. Look for a brand such as Red Boat with no added water, MSG, or preservatives.

Flours (Gluten-Free and Grain-Free)

I am thrilled to include this category of ingredients! When I wrote *The Autoimmune Solution*, autoimmune-approved flours were very difficult to find. With the rise in autoimmunity and our grassroots movement toward wellness, more and more products have come onto the market and even become mainstream. I am so excited that in this cookbook I can provide you with autoimmune-approved recipes for breads, crackers, muffins, pancakes, and even Birthday Cupcakes (page 234)!

Here's a list of gluten-free, grain-free Autoimmune Solution–friendly alternatives to wheat flours. I use them throughout this book for baking or as a coating for chicken, fish, or vegetables. To maintain freshness, store all flours in the refrigerator or freezer once opened. Whatever brand you choose, read the label to make sure that the flour was processed in a gluten-free facility.

Arrowroot Flour Arrowroot is a starch harvested from the rhizome of a tropical herb and has many aliases: arrowroot flour, arrowroot starch, and arrowroot powder. It is most commonly used as a thickener in sauces and soups. Since it's grain-free, arrowroot can be used in baking. Simply whisk together equal parts arrowroot with another grain-free flour substitute, such as cassava. Make sure to whisk arrowroot well to break up any clumps. Arrowroot is available in small spice jars and large packages. I buy it in 1-pound packages to save money.

Cassava Flour Both cassava flour and tapioca flour come from the yucca (also known as mandioca or manioc) root, a staple in many parts of the world. I ate mandioca almost every day for two years while working in rural Paraguay as a Peace Corps volunteer. Cassava flour is made using the entire tuber, which is peeled, dried, and ground. Tapioca flour is produced by washing, pounding, and drying the starchy liquid that remains. Tapioca flour is most frequently diluted with water and used as a thickener in dishes. Cassava flour has the same texture as all-purpose wheat flour or a gluten-free flour blend. This is one of the main flours used in the breakfast and dessert chapters of this book. My favorite is Otto's Naturals cassava flour (see Resources) because the root is peeled and baked, rather than sun-dried, so the flour won't ferment or smell musty.

Coconut Flour Coconut flour is made from dried and ground coconut meat. Like other coconut products, the flour is a good source of lauric acid, a saturated fat thought to support the immune system and the thyroid. For baking, coconut flour is combined with another grain-free flour to provide the best texture.

Tigernut Flour Tigernuts are small, sweet edible tubers that look like striped chickpeas and have been another fantastic addition to my pantry since I wrote *The Autoimmune Solution.* You can purchase them whole to nibble or add them to yogurt, trail mix, and smoothies. They have an almondlike flavor. In addition, tigernuts are high in prebiotic fiber, which is good for feeding good gut bacteria and helping to maintain a healthy gut microbiome (the trillions of microorganisms that live in your digestive tract).

Fruits and Vegetables

A salad of leafy greens, a cup of berries, or a bowl of roasted vegetables provides the best medicine there is. Study after study confirms that eating fruits and vegetables lowers the risk of developing type 2 diabetes, heart

CRUCIFEROUS VEGETABLES: HELPFUL OR HARMFUL?

I am often asked whether people who have Hashimoto's or Graves' diseases or any other form of thyroid dysfunction should avoid cruciferous vegetables (such as broccoli, cauliflower, cabbage, and brussels sprouts), which contain *goitrogens*, which potentially reduce thyroid function. As with any controversial topic, it's best to evaluate the potential risks and benefits yourself. Although studies are inconclusive, I believe that the health-promoting vitamins, minerals, and antioxidants found in cruciferous vegetables far outweigh the minimal potential they have to reduce thyroid function.

If you are worried about cruciferous vegetables and their impact on your thyroid health, I recommend that you cook them, which reduces their goitrogenic properties (however, it also destroys some of their beneficial phytonutrients), and minimize eating them raw (such as in salads and juices). I write much more about this topic and ways to work with your doctor to reverse your Hashimoto's and Graves' in my book *The Thyroid Connection.*

disease, stroke, some cancers, and other conditions. Vegetables in particular provide nourishment, fiber, and satisfaction. When it comes to inflammation, they are gut-healing powerhouses.

It's worth repeating that whenever possible, purchase fresh organic fruits and vegetables or frozen fruits and vegetables without additives. Ask growers at your local farmers' market whether they spray their fruit trees, use genetically modified seeds, or add pesticides. If they do, move on to the next stand. Some farmers may follow organic growing guidelines but can't afford the expense or the time (many years) to become officially certified as organic.

If you are unable to purchase organic produce all the time, once again I recommend that you go to the Environmental Working Group website (www.ewg.org) and review its "Dirty Dozen" and "Clean Fifteen" lists of fruits and vegetables.

For your autoimmune health and wellness, I encourage you to read the list on page 74 of specific fruits and vegetables to enjoy.

Freeze-Dried Fruit The freeze-drying process is a relatively modern preservation process. The fruit is placed on large racks inside of a vacuum chamber. The temperature is lowered to below freezing and then slowly raised. The water in the food moves from a solid state to a gaseous state—maintaining the structure of the food and keeping its nutritional value. The main objective with freeze drying is to remove the moisture so that the food doesn't decompose or grow mold.

Dehydrated Fruit I use dehydrated, or dried, fruit—cranberries, cherries, strawberries—in only a few recipes. Purchase dried fruit without added sugars and preservatives like sulfates. If you're dealing with Candida overgrowth or SIBO, avoid dried fruit and other sugary treats until you have healed these infections.

Herbs

If you have a window with steady sunshine, it's super easy to grow and snip your own parsley, basil, mint, rosemary, and other organic herbs. Or, you can find fresh herbs year-round at supermarkets, farmers' markets, and health food stores. Fresh herbs add flavor to soups, salads, crackers, breads, appetizers, main dishes, and even desserts and smoothies. I recommend using fresh herbs, rather than dried, whenever possible. If you wrap fresh herbs loosely in damp paper towels and store them in the refrigerator, most will last for a week or more. Note that dried herbs are more concentrated than fresh, so if a recipe calls for 1 tablespoon fresh thyme leaves, you will want to use only 1 teaspoon of dried leaves. Additionally, dried herbs can lose their pungency within a few months. Give dried herbs a sniff; if they have no aroma, it's time to replace them.

Meat and Poultry

Bring on those burgers! And pork chops, flank steaks, bone broth, racks of lamb, and roast chickens. The vitamins, minerals, amino acids, and other essential nutrients we need are abundant in organic, grass-fed, pasture-raised meats and poultry. Because they are higher in vitamins and anti-inflammatory fats, these great sources of protein play a starring role when it comes to healing your leaky gut and supporting your immune system.

Conventionally raised, grain-fed cattle are fed an unnatural diet of genetically modified corn and soy. As these crops grew, they were sprayed with pesticides and toxins, and the animals themselves are given antibiotics and engineered growth hormones. This allows the cattle to become supersized—the bigger the animal, the more meat—for market and overtime milk production. The GMO-laden feed given to the cattle affects their gut bacteria, and the toxic chemicals get stored in their fat, so when you eat conventionally raised cattle, you end up eating these harmful substances too. For humans, these growth hormones may increase insulin-like growth factor, which can increase the risk of developing breast, prostate, and other cancers and can affect your hormonal system, including the thyroid gland. So if you must choose between buying organic meat and poultry and buying organic fruits and vegetables, the meat and poultry should win.

Cattle raised on a natural diet of lush, green grass contain higher amounts of the anti-inflammatory omega-3 fatty acids docosahexaenoic acid (DHA) and eicosapentaenoic acid (EPA) and almost five times as much conjugated linoleic acid (CLA). DHA, EPA, and CLA have been shown to support the immune system, help with brain function and mood, boost metabolism, keep cell walls fluid so thyroid hormones can easily enter, and at the same time, reduce inflammation.

Besides growth hormones, cows, chickens, and pigs are also routinely given antibiotics. This leads to antibiotic-resistant supergerms that your body has a difficult time fending off. These antibiotics and supergerms can end up disrupting your endocrine system and can even cause your immune system to go rogue, triggering autoimmunity.

If you don't have a nearby source where you can purchase organic, non-GMO-laden, grass-fed meats, or you simply prefer the convenience of ordering with the click of a mouse, go to ButcherBox.com. This company is one of many that will deliver a monthly shipment of meats right to your door. Butcher Box is committed to raising high-quality 100 percent grass-fed and grass-finished beef; organic, free-range chicken; and heritage breed pork.

Beef When buying beef, look for "100 percent grass-fed, grass-finished" meat, which means that the cows spent their entire lives eating untreated grass. They are not given grain, GMOs, animal by-products, hormones, or antibiotics. One hundred percent grass-fed, pasture-finished cows are harvested anywhere from twenty to thirty months of age, which allows the cattle time to develop the intramuscular fat (marbling) necessary to make the meat a bit less lean while improving its flavor. Cattle (like most people) tend to get fatter as they get older.

"Grass-fed meat" can mean that the cows started their lives eating grass but were then fed a diet of grain during the last three months of their lives to fatten them up. These animals are harvested between eight and twelve months of age. By choosing grass-fed and grass-finished meat you can be certain they are pasture fed their entire life.

Every farmer I have spoken to has said the same thing: consumers should take the time to understand how their meat was raised and

INTERNAL TEMPERATURES FOR MEAT AND POULTRY

Always use a meat thermometer (pages 84 and 306) to test meat and poultry for doneness. Insert the thermometer into the thickest part of the meat. For chicken and turkey, insert the thermometer into the meatiest part of the leg without touching the bone.

Beef, pork, and lamb roasts, steaks, and chops:

Rare: 120–130°F (49–55°C)

Medium rare: 130–135°F (55–57°C)

Medium: 135–145°F (57–63°C)

Medium well: 145–155°F (63–68°C)

Well done: 155°F (68°C)

Chicken and turkey (whole or pieces): 165°F (74°C)

Ground meat: 160°F (71°C)

Pork ribs and shoulders: 190–205°F (88–96°C)

where it comes from. You can also search the internet for a nearby farmer who follows the previously mentioned guidelines and can ship meat packed in dry ice overnight.

Since 100 percent grass-fed and grass-finished animals get more exercise and aren't fed corn and other grains, their beef is naturally leaner, and cooking times are usually shorter, especially when grilling steaks or burgers.

Lamb The same guidelines as for beef apply to purchasing lamb (and other meats): animals must be fully pasture-raised and grass-fed, with no hormones and antibiotics given to them at any time.

Pork Many farmers are now raising rare-breed, heritage pigs, like the Berkshire and Yorkshire varieties. Once weaned, these animals are allowed to roam and forage on grasses and nuts in open pastures. They are bred for flavor rather than leanness, so their juicy meat has more intramuscular fat. Look for 100 percent pasture-raised pork at farmers' markets and online at ButcherBox.com.

Chicken and Turkey To be called "organic," chickens and turkeys must be fed organic food (grown without pesticides or the use of GMOs), receive no antibiotics and hormones, and be allowed to wander outdoors.

Mustard

I love the zing that mustard adds to dishes. Whenever I smell Dijon mustard, I am reminded of my mom because it was one of her favorite condiments. She was famous for her amazing salads and salad dressings. We used to joke that she had been a rabbit in another lifetime because of how many salads and greens she ate every day. I carry on Mom's salad legacy with my own family by making a large salad for dinner almost every night. Mom's famous salad dressing recipe with Dijon mustard—Betty's Italian Dressing— can be found on page 205. Be sure to use an organic brand of Dijon mustard made with mustard seeds, apple cider vinegar, and seasonings. Avoid those made with white wine.

Protein Powders, Collagen Protein, and Gelatin

The Myers Way is about supporting, rather than suppressing, the immune system. To do this, we need to eat foods that help build and repair the body's tissues, including the nine essential amino acids found in complete proteins. They are deemed "essential" because your body can't synthesize them on its own, meaning you must get them from your diet. These all-important amino acids help build and repair every single structure in your body, which requires a great deal of dietary protein every day in order to be done correctly and efficiently.

And yet time and time again, through nutritional testing I find that many of my patients—especially vegetarians and vegans—are deficient in these essential amino acids. I was a vegetarian for twenty-seven years, and

I believe that my nutritional deficiency as a result of my diet is one of the reasons I developed Graves' disease.

Many of the protein powders on the market contain gluten, dairy (whey), grains, eggs, legumes such as genetically modified soybeans, and sugar as well as solvents and other inflammatory ingredients that are not good for anyone, especially those of us looking to support rather than wreck our immune systems. After going five years without a smoothie, I decided to formulate my own autoimmune-friendly protein powder, The Myers Way Paleo Protein®, which is sourced from 100 percent grass-fed beef that was never given GMOs, antibiotics, or hormones.

The Myers Way Paleo Protein doesn't contain gluten, dairy, grains, eggs, legumes, or sugars. Everyone can use it, whether they are following an autoimmune protocol, avoiding inflammatory foods, or just looking to enjoy a rich, creamy, and healthy smoothie. Children and adults alike love smoothies that include this protein powder, and you'll find several in this book.

Collagen protein, on the other hand, is an incomplete protein because it doesn't contain all nine essential amino acids; however, it is very rich in four key amino acids that are often lacking in our modern diets. Your body can produce collagen, but it requires specific amino acids, adequate vitamin C, healthy fibroblasts (the cells that make collagen), and more. Furthermore, your production of collagen rapidly declines as you age, which is bad news because collagen is the glue that holds your body together. Your skin, gut barrier, bones, connective tissue, cartilage, and joints all depend on ample collagen to be healthy, strong, and flexible. The good news is you can easily increase your collagen in order to maintain a healthy gut, healthy bones and joints, and beautiful hair, skin, and nails! Gut-Healing Bone Broth (page 71) is a great source of collagen, however you would need to drink a lot of it every day to even come close to maintaining enough collagen as you age, and that isn't always feasible or convenient. That's why collagen powder has become enormously popular.

It's encouraging that more people are aware of the gut-repairing and other body-boosting benefits of collagen, however, many of the collagen powders on the market don't contain the required amino acids that give collagen its health benefits. In addition, many collagen products on the market are not sourced from organic and pasture-raised animals, and are overprocessed and denatured by high heat, destroying the delicate peptides contained within.

Because I know the healing benefits of collagen and I like to enjoy it at least once a day, whether in my morning smoothie or evening Gut-Soothing Collagen Tea (page 126) (or both!), I sourced my own collagen protein. The Myers Way Collagen Protein comes from 100 percent grass-fed cows that are never given antibiotics, hormones, or GMO-laden feed. It is pure type I and III collagen. These types of collagen are the most abundant in the body and provide all the benefits to your gut health, skin, bones, hair, nails, and connective tissues. They contain important amino acids and peptides that help prevent and repair leaky gut, which is key for anyone with auto-immunity or an inflammatory condition.

The Myers Way Collagen Protein is tasteless and dissolves instantly, so you can easily add it to any liquid and you'll never know the difference. To make sure you're getting enough collagen protein, simply add a tablespoon of it to smoothies, teas, mocktails, or soups for an extra gut-healing, protein boost.

The Myers Way Gelatin has all of the same amino acids and health benefits as collagen, with a different chemical structure that makes it in-dispensable in baked goods. Gelatin has a gel-like quality that acts as a binding agent in place of eggs in recipes. The Myers Way Gelatin also comes from 100 percent grass-fed cows that are never given antibiotics, hormones, or GMO-laden feed, and it is colorless and flavorless. Unlike collagen, however, The Myers Way Gelatin thickens whatever you add it to, so you'll want to use it in baked goods, gummy snacks, sauces, and soups and stick with The Myers Way Collagen Protein for smoothies, teas, and other beverages.

Seafood: Fish and Shellfish

When it comes to seafood, take a walk on the wild side and purchase fish that is labeled "wild" or "wild-caught." They're better for your body and taste better than farmed varieties. Wild fish eat a natural diet and live in open waters. Go for wild-caught salmon, halibut, sardines, cod, and shrimp. Eat them fresh or freeze them in serving portions for another day.

"Farmed" fish are raised in enormous pens and fed a limited diet of pellets that contain corn, grains, and ground-up wild fish as well as antibiotics, pesticides, and artificial coloring to make their flesh look like that of wild fish. Diseases run rampant among fish packed into these pens. If they escape, they eat and contaminate schools of wild fish. Farmed-raised fish are notoriously contaminated with polychlorinated biphenyls (PCBs), toxic chemicals that disrupt our endocrine systems, including the thyroid. Avoid farmed tilapia, sea bass, salmon, and shrimp.

Salmon is the most popular fish in North America, so it's important to know the differences between farmed and wild salmon. Farmed salmon has wide white fat bands throughout the flesh, while wild salmon is generally darker and has thinner fat bands. Don't be fooled by color; farmed salmon are fed food coloring to make them look like naturally pink wild salmon.

Most canned salmon is wild-caught, but check the label to be sure. Alaskan pink or sockeye salmon is always wild-caught. If the label says "Atlantic" salmon, it's farmed and may contain PCBs, which contaminate soil, rivers, and lakes. My trusted source for wild-caught fresh and canned seafood is www.Vitalchoice.com (see Resources).

Shrimp runs a close second behind salmon when it comes to popularity. Any peeled, deveined, cooked, or frozen shrimp is exempt from "country of origin" and "farm versus wild" labeling. Most imported shrimp is farmed in tanks or enormous industrial ponds, where chemicals and waste can cause illness and decay. They're also treated with preservatives.

When shopping for shrimp, know that labeling can be meaningless. Even the seller may not know where the shrimp come from. When possible, buy wild American shrimp caught off the Gulf and South Atlantic coasts. You can order them online from www.Vitalchoice.com.

Overfishing, pollution, and climate change have resulted in a shortage of edible, wild fish and shellfish. And the US Department of Agriculture (USDA) has no organic standards for seafood. To help you choose the best seafood, I recommend visiting the highly respected Monterey Bay Aquarium Seafood Watch at www.seafoodwatch.org. Type in the name of your favorite anti-inflammatory seafood and three categories of your choice will pop up telling you which ones are Best (green) or Good (yellow) to consume and which ones to Avoid (red). A free app offers the latest recommendations for buying and cooking sustainable seafood and making sushi.

Seaweed

Seaweed, or sea vegetables harvested from marine waters, are loaded with iodine, which is essential for supporting your thyroid gland, especially if you have autoimmune thyroid disease. Seaweed is also rich in the omega-3 fatty acid DHA, which is very anti-inflammatory and supports brain function, vision, cell wall integrity, and the central nervous system. Seaweed is just what your thyroid gland ordered. Use nori for vegetable and seafood rolls, salads, and soups. Wakame can be soaked and added to salads and soups. Never harvest your own seaweed; the waters may be polluted.

Spices

Herbs and spices add flavor and bring dishes alive, as well; they also contain important healing and anti-inflammatory properties. Purchase organic spices in bulk quantities and then transfer them to dark glass containers away from light and heat so they last longer. Ground herbs will keep for six months to a year. Give them a sniff them before using them; if you can't smell them, it's time to replace them.

Black and White Pepper The peppercorn, despite its name, is not in the nightshade family, so feel free to use it to season your food. Black and white peppercorns are grown in India and come from the same vine, but they are harvested at different times. Black ones are picked when they are still green and then dried in the sun until they become wrinkled and black. The best are Tellicherry peppercorns. They are available everywhere.

White peppercorns—though they're actually creamy in color—are allowed to ripen on the vine for a longer period of time. Their hulls are removed before they are dried. They are a bit spicier than black peppercorns, and some cooks prefer to use them on light-colored dishes for aesthetic reasons.

Whichever color you choose, use a peppermill to freshly grind pepper as needed. The preground stuff is dusty and flavorless. Cayenne pepper comes from the nightshade family, so you should avoid it.

Ginger This is my absolute favorite spice, probably because it reminds me of my mom. When I was growing up, she always cooked everything from scratch, including her famous ginger snap and molasses-ginger cookies—I didn't know that chocolate-chip cookies existed until I attended school.

In my kitchen, you'll find fresh, whole gingerroot as well as grated gingerroot in my refrigerator, ground ginger in my cabinet, and ginger teas in my pantry. Although we call it "gingerroot," it's actually a rhizome like turmeric. Use a knife or vegetable peeler to remove the outer skin, then slice or grate the ginger using a microplane zester. Many recipes in this cookbook include ginger. I am thrilled that my favorite spice works similarly to turmeric to reduce inflammation and, in some studies, has been shown to reduce pain associated with arthritis.

Lemongrass This is my second favorite spice. My dad was a political science professor, with a focus in Asian studies. We often hosted Chinese graduate students at our home, and to thank us, they would cook traditional Chinese dishes for us that often included lemongrass. The best way to cook with lemongrass is to first remove the tough, outer leaves and then mince or puree the bulb at the bottom of the stem to make marinades, dressings, and stir-fried dishes. You can steep the leaves in hot water for tea. To freeze fresh lemongrass, store thinly sliced pieces in single layers in a small glass jar. To dry leaves, bundle them and hang them upside down in a dark place until dry, then store them in tightly sealed jars. Buy fresh lemongrass, which you can find at many grocery stores and Asian markets; dried lemongrass doesn't have the fragrant scent of fresh and is not as flavorful.

Sea Salt True sea salt is simply the solid crystals left behind once seawater is evaporated, which makes its taste and texture briny and clean. Sea salts taste unique and have different amounts of essential minerals depending on where the seawater comes from.

Table and kosher salts contain additives or preservatives, because mined salt is refined by heating it to more than 2,000°F. As a result, essential trace minerals disappear during processing. An anticaking agent is then added to make the salt flow freely, but it turns purple. To make it snow white and appealing to consumers, the salt is bleached, and glucose, talcum, and aluminum silicate are added back in. Coarse kosher salt is refined in the same way, but iodine isn't added at the end.

A pinch or two of pure sea salt enhances food, rather than making it salty. Sea salts come in a wide range of colors—from pink and pale gray to deep beige, depending on where the water comes from—and a range of textures, from fine to coarse. It's available in grocery stores everywhere and online. Always read the label to make sure the sea salt is pure.

Turmeric This is the superstar of the spice world. If you're unfamiliar with turmeric, allow me to introduce you. Turmeric is a rhizome, or a rootlike stem, native to India. With a pungent flavor and bright reddish-orange flesh, turmeric is widely used in cooking and as a medicine throughout the world. It adds a warm, earthy aroma and flavor to all kinds of dishes, especially curries.

Curcumin, which causes the orange pigment in turmeric, is a potent antioxidant with loads of health benefits. Turmeric is chock-full of beneficial compounds, including carotenoids, curcuminoids, and essential oils called turmerones. What's so great about the curcumin in turmeric? It helps modulate your body's inflammation response, fight free radicals, encourage a balanced and healthy immune response, support gut lining and intestinal health, promote detox pathways, and support liver function.

Curcumin is best absorbed when consumed with fat such as the coconut milk found in my Golden Milk recipe (page 120). Studies have shown that to receive the full benefits of curcumin, you would need to consume very large quantities of it. For that reason, I recommend that people with autoimmunity supplement their diets with a fat-soluble form of curcumin (see chapter 18 for more information on supplements).

Ground turmeric is widely available in bulk, and fresh turmeric, which can be grated using a microplane zester, is becoming more available. (Know that fresh turmeric will turn your hands and cutting board bright orange!) Whole fresh turmeric is sold at many grocery stores, farmers' markets, and places that carry products from India.

Sweeteners

I've included a few sweetener options here that are not found in *The Autoimmune Solution*. Because many of you have already gone through the thirty-day protocol and regained your health, you may be ready to add these in on special occasions, as I have done myself. If you're new to The Myers Way, you're still working to eliminate your symptoms, or you're currently experiencing or treating Candida overgrowth or SIBO, you can substitute or skip these ingredients until you've healed. (Learn more about Candida and SIBO on page 25.) Then, as you move down the autoimmune spectrum from high inflammation to low or no inflammation (see page 21) and are living symptom-free, you can allow yourself to celebrate, branch out, and enjoy the occasional indulgence of dried fruit, honey, maple syrup, and sweeteners used in some of the recipes in this book.

Coconut Sugar Coconut sugar is made from boiled and rehydrated sap of the coconut palm. It looks very similar to brown sugar. Although natural coconut sugar contains less glucose and fructose than cane sugar, you should still use it in moderation.

Honey Be sure to always use raw honey (except children younger than twelve months), which bees make from the nectar of flowers. It is pure, unfiltered, and unpasteurized. Most of the honey consumed today is pasteurized, which means it has been heated and filtered. This robs it of its incredible nutritional value and healing powers. A tablespoon or two of raw honey adds antimicrobial and immune-boosting properties as well as improving seasonal allergies.

Maple Syrup This all-American natural sweetener contains significant amounts of zinc and manganese, which are important minerals, especially for those people with inflammation. Unrefined maple syrup has higher levels of beneficial nutrients, antioxidants, and phytochemicals than refined sugars. When the sap of certain maple trees is boiled and reduced, the result is maple syrup. The darker the color, the stronger the flavor. Be sure to buy "pure maple syrup," not pancake syrup, which contains maple syrup flavoring and preservatives. It takes 40 gallons of sap to make 1 gallon of syrup, which is why pure maple syrup costs more; however, a little bit of the real thing goes a long way.

Molasses I had fun making molasses with my Paraguayan family while serving as a Peace Corps volunteer. I helped cut the sugar cane using a machete (it was much harder than it looked!), removed the outer leaves, and ran the stalk though a hand-cranked press to extract the "sugar" or juice. The juice was then boiled several times to make the molasses. Each time it was boiled the molasses became darker and thicker. Unlike highly refined sugars, molasses contains significant amounts of vitamin B6 and minerals, including calcium, magnesium, iron, and manganese, all of which are great in supporting your immune system. Blackstrap molasses, which comes from the third boil, is also a good source of potassium.

Stevia Stevia is an all-natural sweetener and sugar substitute extracted from the leaves of the *Stevia rebaudiana* plant that is indigenous to South America. The Guaraní people have been using it as a sweetener and medicine for more than fifteen hundred years. Also, during my time in Paraguay, I helped farmers grow and export stevia to the United States and Japan.

The active compounds of stevia are steviol glycosides, which are estimated to be 150 to 300 times sweeter than sugar and don't raise blood glucose levels. With stevia, a little bit goes a long way. I recommend purchasing 100 percent organic stevia in powdered leaf form or a 100 percent liquid extract. Brands such as Truvia and Pure Via are not pure stevia, rather they are stevia mixed with sugar alcohols and natural flavors and other added chemicals.

Vinegar

You will see apple cider vinegar used often in this cookbook. I recommend that you use a brand that is organic and made without yeast, such as Bragg (see Resources). Most other apple cider vinegars on the market are made from apples that are fermented with yeast. (Yeast is not approved on *The Autoimmune Solution* thirty-day protocol.)

These are a handful of recipes for staples that I use frequently. To save time, keep some Gut-Healing Bone Broth, Cauliflower Rice, Coconut Milk, caramelized onions, and other basics in the refrigerator or freezer.

Cauliflower Rice

Makes about 4 cups

Although you can find packages of cauliflower rice in many markets these days, it's easy to make your own and so much less expensive. There are two ways to make cauliflower rice—on the stovetop or in the oven. In addition to using it in my recipes, you can combine cauliflower rice with sautéed onions, shallots, and/or garlic for a simple side dish. Add fresh herbs and seasonings such as cilantro and lime.

1 head cauliflower, pulled apart into 1- to 2-inch florets

Rinse the florets in a colander and shake off excess water. (You can also give them a whirl in a salad spinner to dry them.)

Place cauliflower in a food processor or blender. (You can also rice the cauliflower using a box grater. Be sure to watch your knuckles! Using a blender will result in uneven "grains.") Depending on the size of your machine, you may have to do this in two or three batches. Pulse the cauliflower three or four times until it looks like rice. Store it in a glass container in the refrigerator for up to 2 or 3 days or freeze up to 1 month.

For stovetop rice: Heat 1 or 2 tablespoons avocado oil in a large skillet over medium-high heat. Add the cauliflower rice and a bit of sea salt and black pepper, to taste. Cook, stirring frequently, until the rice is lightly brown and cooked through (taste a few kernels to check).

For oven-roasted rice: Heat oven to 425°F. Spread cauliflower rice on a sheet pan and season with salt and pepper, to taste. Roast, stirring occasionally, for 15 to 20 minutes (or longer if you want it darker).

Coconut Milk

Makes about 4 cups

It can be hard to find canned coconut milk without all of the added ingredients such as sugars and gums. You can easily make your own.

1 8-ounce package unsweetened, shredded coconut

4 cups hot water

Put coconut in a blender. Pour water on top of coconut. Let mixture sit for a few minutes to soften the coconut. Blend on high for 1 minute.

Pour mixture into a bowl through a fine-mesh sieve or a nut milk bag (available in health food stores or online). Push through the sieve or squeeze the bag to remove as much milk as possible from the coconut. Use immediately or pour into a glass jar and refrigerate for 3 to 4 days.

Coconut Butter

I use a lot of coconut butter, which can be costly if you buy it, so I make it myself. All you need is unsweetened shredded coconut and a food processor or high-speed blender. Try the flavored variations, too.

3 cups unsweetened, shredded coconut

Put the coconut in a food processor or blender and process for 30 seconds. Stop the machine and, using a spatula, scrape down the sides. Repeat this step several times until the coconut releases its oils and the mixture becomes smooth and creamy. If desired, add one of the flavorings listed below.

Scrape the butter into a jar and refrigerate. Before using, let the coconut butter come to room temperature or set the jar in a bowl of hot water.

Chocolate Coconut Butter: Add 2 tablespoons cocoa powder to the food processor or blender.

Cinnamon Coconut Butter: Add 1 teaspoon maple syrup and ½ teaspoon ground cinnamon to the food processor or blender.

Peppermint Coconut Butter: Add 1 to 2 drops essential peppermint oil to the food processor or blender.

Pumpkin Spice: Add 2 tablespoons pumpkin puree, ¼ teaspoon ground cinnamon, ¼ teaspoon ground ginger, ⅛ teaspoon ground nutmeg, and ⅛ teaspoon ground cloves to the food processor or blender.

Toasted Coconut Butter: Heat oven to 325°F. Arrange the coconut on a parchment paper–lined baking sheet. Bake for 3 to 5 minutes, then gently stir. Bake for an additional 3 to 5 minutes, watching carefully so the coconut doesn't burn. Remove from the oven and add to the food processor or blender.

Coconut Milk Yogurt

Makes 2 servings

Coconut cream (the top layer in canned coconut milk) is what makes this yogurt rich and decadent. This is used as the base for Tzatziki (page 204) and can be made as plain or flavored.

2 13½-ounce cans full-fat coconut milk, refrigerated overnight

2 capsules 100 billion CFU probiotics (see chapter 18)

1 tablespoon tapioca starch (optional)

Use a spoon to remove the top creamy layer from both cans of coconut milk and place into a small bowl. Save the thinner liquid for another use. Empty the contents of one probiotic capsule into the coconut cream and whisk together. Discard the capsule. If using the tapioca starch to thicken the yogurt, add to coconut cream mixture and whisk again.

Pour into a 16-ounce glass jar and cover with a lid. Place the jar in an unheated oven for 18 to 24 hours. The mixture will become thicker and develop a "tangy" yogurt flavor. Put the jar in the refrigerator to stop fermentation. Refrigerate and consume within 2 weeks.

Vanilla Coconut Yogurt: Add 2 teaspoons pure vanilla extract and ½ teaspoon stevia.

Cinnamon Swirl Yogurt: Add 2 teaspoons ground cinnamon and ½ teaspoon stevia.

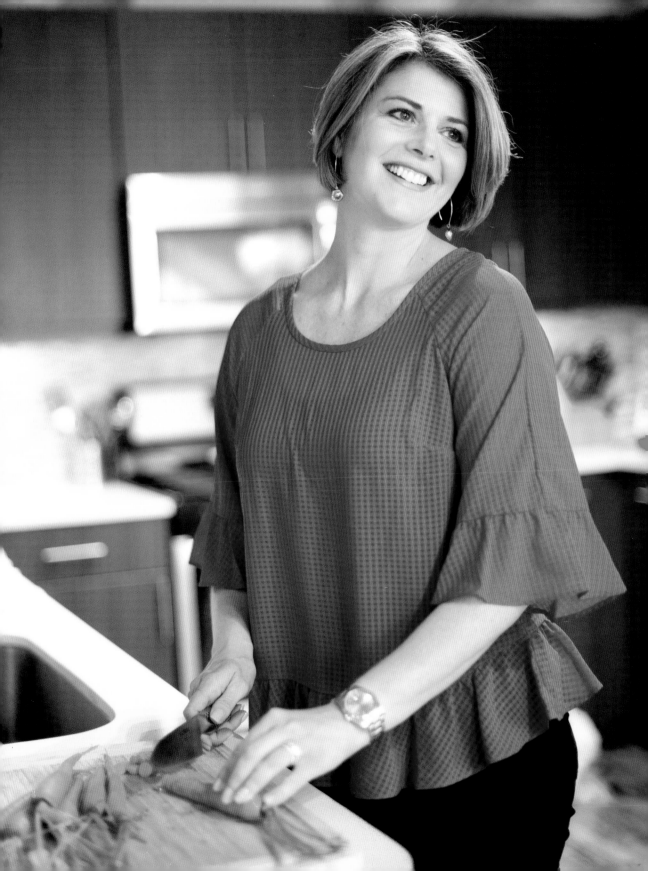

Tigernut Waffles, page 95

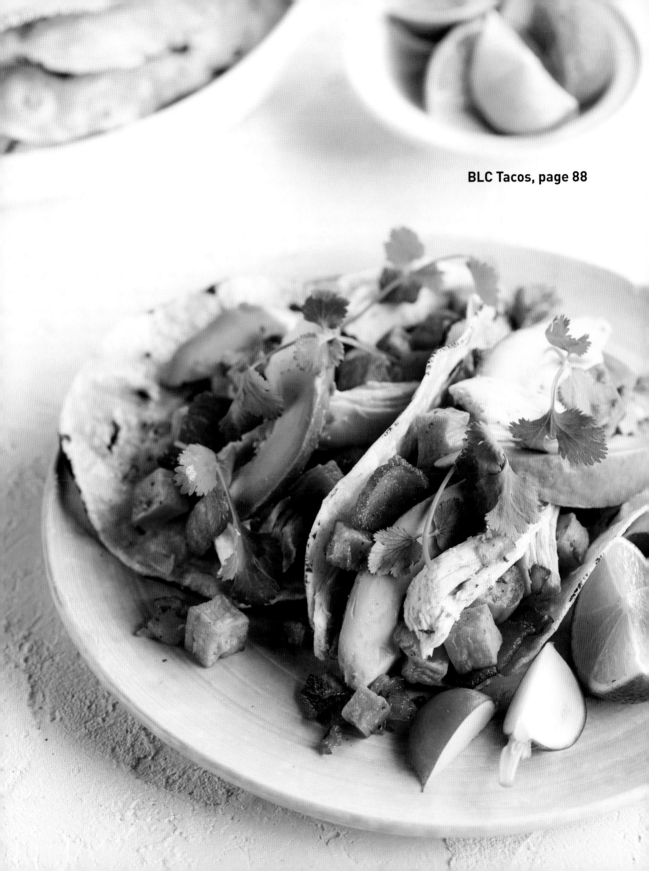
BLC Tacos, page 88

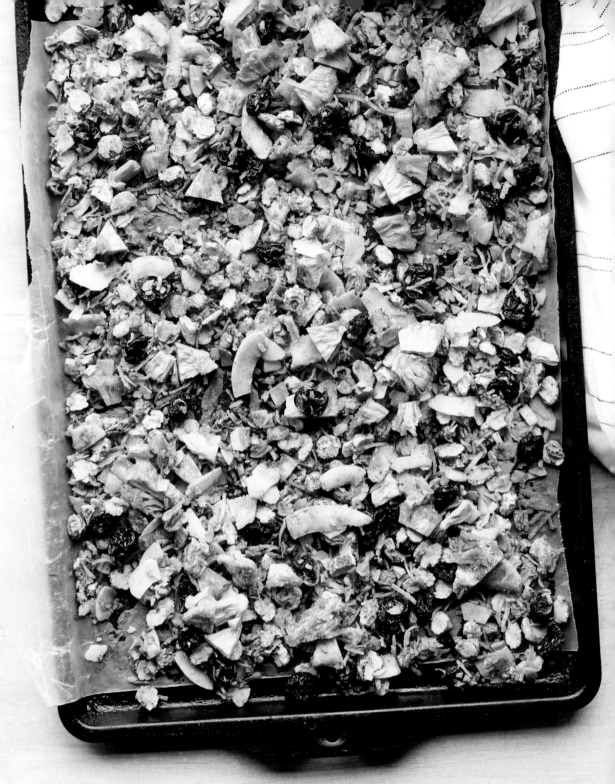

Crunchy Maple Granola, page 94

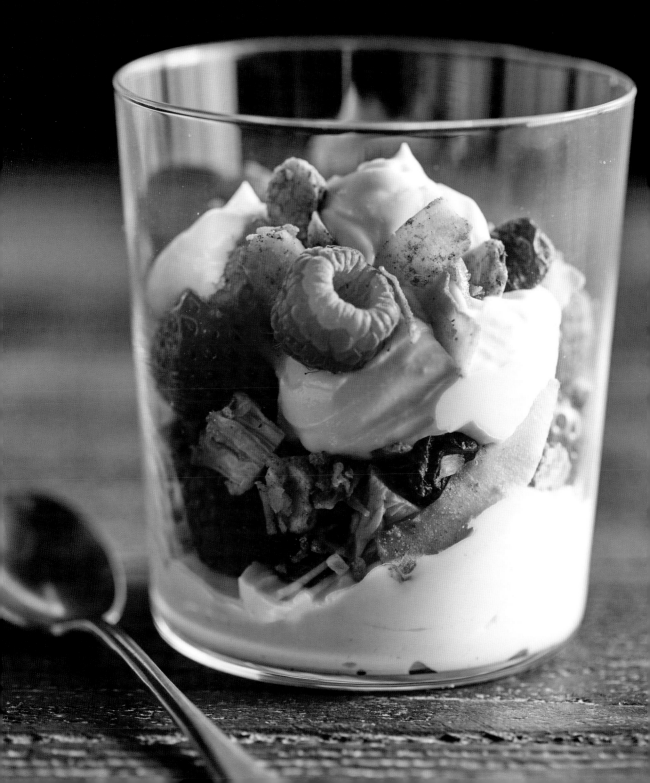

Coconut Yogurt Parfaits, page 101

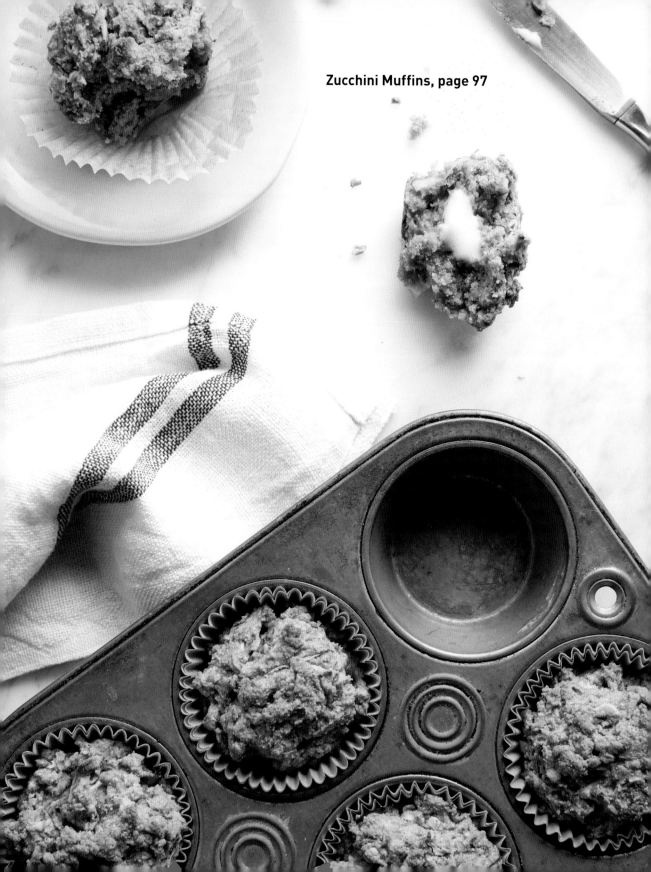

Zucchini Muffins, page 97

Golden Milk, page 120

Gut-Healing Bone Broth, page 71

Gut-Healing Bone Broth

Makes 8 cups

Gut-Healing Bone Broth is used as the base of many of the soup recipes in this book. The nutrients in bone broth work to heal the mucosal lining of the digestive tract, to reduce inflammation, and to promote sleep and a calm mind—all great benefits for your thyroid and immune system. In addition, I recommend savoring this broth in the morning served in your favorite mug. If you find yourself with some extra after 3 or 4 days, freeze the leftovers in small glass containers to enjoy later.

1 organic, pasture-raised leftover chicken carcass *or* 1 pound organic, pasture-raised chicken parts, such as wings and thighs *or* 1 pound pastured beef bones, knuckle, neck, and marrow

2 tablespoons apple cider vinegar

1 teaspoon sea salt

2 garlic cloves, peeled and smashed with the flat side of a knife

1 cup chopped carrots, celery, and onions (optional)

8 cups filtered water (or as needed)

Put the chicken carcass or beef bones in a slow cooker with the vinegar, salt, garlic, and vegetables, if using. Add enough water to cover the bones.

Set the slow cooker to low and cook for 8 to 24 hours (the longer you cook, the more gelatin or collagen you draw out of the bones, giving you more gut-healing properties).

When the broth is done (begins to gel at the top or has been cooked for desired length of time), use a slotted spoon to remove the bones. Pour broth into a large saucepan through a fine-mesh strainer. Refrigerate up to 4 days. Before reheating, use a spoon to scrape off the surface fat. Or, freeze individual portions up to 2 months.

Onions

Onions just need a little heat and a bit of fat—bacon drippings, avocado oil, or coconut oil—to bring out their natural sweetness. Here are a few guidelines for cooking yellow, sweet, white, or red onions to three stages of doneness. They may need more or less cooking time, depending on the size of your skillet (a wider one is best), the kind of fat you use, and the heat level (low and slow is best). A huge pile of sliced or chopped onions will reduce significantly, so make a big batch. Refrigerate cooked onions for 5 days or freeze for 1 month.

Chop, dice, or slice onions and cook in a wide skillet over low heat with a little fat:

Soft Onions: For 3 to 5 minutes.

Translucent Onions: For 5 to 7 minutes, until they become paler in color.

Caramelized Onions: For 25 to 30 minutes, stirring frequently to prevent burning, until deep brown in color and meltingly soft. The onions, like mushrooms, will release a little water that will eventually evaporate.

Garlic

When beginning a recipe with oil and garlic, put both in a cold skillet, then turn on the heat to medium. Stir the garlic and cook just until you can smell it, then add the next ingredients. Be careful, as whole garlic cloves or sliced, minced, or grated garlic can burn quickly and become bitter, ruining your dish.

To roast garlic: Heat oven to 400°F. Cut the top, not the root end, off of a whole garlic bulb. Place the bulb cut side down on a small parchment-lined baking sheet and roast until the garlic can be pierced with a knife, about 20 to 30 minutes, depending on the size of the garlic. Let the garlic sit until it's cool enough to handle, and then squeeze out the garlic cloves and discard the papery skin. You can roast several bulbs at one time. Refrigerate them in a covered glass container for 2 to 3 days.

Foods to Enjoy

Quality Proteins

- Bone broth
- Organic, grass-fed beef
- Organic, grass-fed lamb
- Organic pork or bacon
- Organic, pasture-raised poultry (chicken, duck, turkey)
- Organ meats (heart, liver, marrow, kidney, sweetbreads)
- Sardines
- The Myers Way Protein
- The Myers Way Collagen Protein
- The Myers Way Gelatin
- Wild-caught fresh fish (cod, halibut, haddock, salmon, pollock, snapper, sole, trout)
- Wild-caught shrimp
- Wild game

Organic Nonstarchy Vegetables

- Alfalfa sprouts (also broccoli, radish, and sunflower sprouts)
- Artichokes
- Arugula*
- Asparagus
- Avocados
- Bamboo shoots
- Bean sprouts
- Bok choy*
- Broccoli*
- Broccolini (or rapini, or broccoli raab)
- Brussels sprouts*
- Cabbage*
- Cauliflower*
- Celery
- Cucumbers
- Fennel
- Garlic
- Green onions
- Greens* (beet, collard, dandelion, kale, mustard, turnip)
- Hearts of palm
- Herbs (parsley, cilantro, basil, rosemary, thyme, dill, lemongrass, etc.)
- Kohlrabi
- Leeks
- Lettuce (endive, escarole, baby lettuces, Bibb, butter, romaine, iceberg)
- Mushrooms
- Okra
- Olives
- Onions
- Purslane
- Radishes*
- Rhubarb
- Sauerkraut
- Scallions
- Shallots
- Spinach
- Summer squash
- Swiss chard
- Watercress
- Zucchini

*These are foods that it is suggested to eat cooked rather than raw for those with thyroid conditions

Starchy Vegetables

- Beets
- Carrots
- Cassava, cassava flour
- Chestnuts
- Jerusalem artichokes
- Jicama
- Parsnips
- Plantains, plantain flour
- Pumpkins
- Rutabagas
- Sweet potatoes, sweet potato flour
- Taro
- Tigernuts, tigernut flour
- Turnips
- Water chestnuts
- Yams
- Yucca

Healthy Fats

- Avocado, avocado oil
- Coconut, coconut oil, coconut flour, coconut butter/manna/milk/yogurt/cream
- Ghee (if you tolerate it)
- Grapeseed oil
- Olives, olive oil
- Flaxseed oil
- Animal fat (lard, beef tallow)
- Palm oil

Organic Fruits

- Apples
- Apricots
- Bananas
- Bilberries
- Blackberries
- Blueberries
- Boysenberries
- Currants
- Cherries
- Cranberries
- Dates (limit during the thirty-day protocol and avoid if treating Candida overgrowth or SIBO)
- Dragonfruit
- Elderberries
- Figs
- Gooseberries
- Grapefruit
- Grapes
- Guavas
- Huckleberries
- Kiwis
- Kumquats
- Lemons
- Limes
- Loquats
- Lychees
- Mangos
- Melons (cantaloupe, honeydew, watermelon, etc.)
- Mulberries
- Nectarines
- Papayas
- Passionfruit
- Peaches
- Pears
- Persimmons
- Pineapples
- Plums
- Pomegranates
- Quince
- Raisins (limit during the thirty-day protocol and avoid if treating Candida overgrowth or SIBO)
- Raspberries
- Star fruit
- Strawberries
- Tamarillos
- Tamarind fruit

Flours

- Arrowroot starch
- Cassava flour
- Coconut flour
- Plantain flour
- Sweet potato flour
- Tapioca flour
- Tigernut flour

Dairy Alternative

- Camel's milk[†]
- Coconut milk, yogurt, cream
- Tigernut milk

Flavorful Seasonings and Condiments

- Anise
- Apple cider vinegar
- Basil
- Bay leaf
- Cacao
- Cilantro/coriander
- Cinnamon
- Cloves
- Cumin
- Dill
- Garlic
- Ginger
- Ground black pepper
- Mint
- Nutmeg
- Oregano
- Parsley
- Rosemary
- Sea salt
- Stevia
- Tarragon
- Thyme
- Turmeric
- Vanilla

Beverages

- Bone broth
- Coconut milk
- Fruit and vegetable juices, unsweetened
- Smoothies
- Mocktails
- Tea, herbal, caffeine-free
- Tigernut milk
- Water, filtered or sparkling

[†]The proteins in camel's milk are very different than cow, sheep, or goat dairy. I find most people can tolerate them well. If you are concerned about including, follow instructions in chapter 17 on how to reintroduce foods.

Foods to Toss

Toxic Foods

- Alcohol
- Fast foods, junk foods, processed foods
- Food additives: any foods that contain artificial colors, flavors, or preservatives
- Genetically modified foods (GMOs), including canola oil and beet sugar
- Processed meats: canned meats (such as SPAM; canned fish is okay), cold cuts, hotdogs
- Processed and refined oils: mayonnaise, salad dressings, shortening, spreads
- Refined oils, hydrogenated fats, *trans* fats, including margarine
- Stimulants and caffeine: coffee, yerba mate
- Sweeteners: sugar, sugar alcohols, sweetened juices, high-fructose corn syrup
- *Trans* fats and hydrogenated oils (frequently found in packaged and processed foods)

Inflammatory Foods

- Corn and anything made from corn or containing high-fructose corn syrup
- Dairy, including cow, sheep and goat milk‡ cheese, cottage cheese, cream, yogurt, butter, ice cream, frozen yogurt, and nondairy creamers, whey protein, casein
- Eggs: chicken and duck§
- Gluten: anything that contains spelt, barley, rye, or wheat
- Gluten-free grains and pseudograins: amaranth, buckwheat, millet, oats, quinoa, rice
- Legumes: beans, green beans, garbanzos, lentils, peas, snow peas, peanuts, and soy
- Nightshades: eggplant, peppers, potatoes, tomatoes
- Nuts: including nut butters
- Peanuts
- Seeds: including seed butters
- Soy: (miso, tofu, tempeh, soy milk, soy creamer, soy yogurt, soy cheese, kimchi)

‡Though the proteins in sheep and goat's milk are different, some people may not tolerate them. After thirty-day protocol, follow instructions in chapter 17 on how to reintroduce foods.

§Though the proteins in duck eggs are different, some people may not tolerate them. After thirty-day protocol, follow instructions in chapter 17 on how to reintroduce foods.

OCCASIONAL FOODS

As part of following The Myers Way for life, I have incorporated some cacao and natural sweeteners (such as honey, maple syrup, molasses, and coconut palm sugar) into some of the recipes. Enjoy these in moderation.

Kitchen Tools

Everyone needs to make wise choices when it comes to choosing pots, pans, storage containers, wrappers, and anything else that comes in contact with our food. Whenever possible, choose glass over plastic for food storage and mixing. Choose wooden or stainless-steel utensils over plastic for mixing ingredients. This guide will help you make other informed decisions (also see Resources).

Cookware

Tame the Toxins is the third pillar of The Myers Way, so choosing toxin-free cookware is just as important as choosing the food you cook in it. Cast-iron cookware is nontoxic and one of my favorite kinds of cookware. Where I'm from in the South, people pass along their cast-iron skillets and Dutch ovens from one generation to the next. Investing in two or three pieces of quality cookware described below will improve your cooking and reduce your toxic burden.

Healthy Cookware to Purchase

Enameled Cast-Iron skillets, pans, baking dishes, and Dutch ovens are easy to care for and available in many colors. If you want the benefits of iron, then opt for non-enameled coated cast-iron cookware.

Recommended enameled cast-iron brands include Le Creuset, Staub, and Lodge (see Resources).

Cast-Iron Cookware is more affordable than enameled cast-iron cookware and ideal for cooking. Cast iron can be used on a cooktop or grill or in the oven. Although some pots and pans are said to be "preseasoned," they can all benefit from some extra care. To season a cast-iron pan, heat it on the stovetop until it is smoking hot; then, using a paper towel, rub a little bacon lard or avocado, coconut, or olive oil on the interior surface. Turn the heat off and let it cool. Repeat this process two or three times, and your new cookware is ready to use. The more you use a cast-iron skillet, the more seasoned it will become. An added benefit of cast-iron cookware is that small amounts of iron will be released while you cook your food. This can be helpful for people with thyroid dysfunction and iron deficiency who need to increase their intake of iron.

Stainless-Steel Cookware is affordable and very stable at high temperatures. This cookware is lighter than cast-iron, resistant to scratching, and lasts significantly longer than coated cookware. However, since stainless steel is not nonstick, you will need to use more oil or fat when cooking.

Glass Cookware. Glass baking dishes, casseroles with lids, measuring cups, and bowls come in many sizes and shapes. Glass is a sturdy material that will not release chemicals or toxic metals into your food. Glass dishes are ideal for mixing, baking, and storing leftovers. I recommend using glass storage containers instead of plastic ones in order to avoid toxins like bisphenol-A (BPA), which can disrupt your endocrine system and thyroid hormones.

Toxic Cookware to Toss

Ceramic-Coated Pans are made with various metals coated with a synthetic polymer that is softer than metal. Once the coating starts to wear off, toxic metals can leach into your cooked food, depending on the material underneath the coating.

Nonstick Cookware (such as Teflon) contains a synthetic coating of polytetrafluoroethylene (PTFE), a plastic polymer that can release harmful and carcinogenic gases at temperatures exceeding 500°F. In humans, these fumes can cause flu-like symptoms several hours after exposure, resulting in a condition called *polymer fume fever* that is often misdiagnosed as a viral flu. The gases are so toxic that they are fatal for most birds.

Aluminum Cookware is often coated to prevent aluminum leaching from the cookware. These coatings can chip and wear off easily. Aluminum cookware can be affordable, but the risk of aluminum leaching into your food and contributing to a potential aluminum toxicity isn't worth it. Aluminum can accumulate in your brain, lungs, bones, and other tissues, causing tangles in nerve fibers and leading to muscular dysfunction and memory loss. While aluminum has not been shown to be a cause of Alzheimer's disease, increased levels of aluminum in the brain have been noted in autopsies of Alzheimer's patients, which suggests that aluminum toxicity may be a risk factor. Other sources of aluminum to be avoided include aluminum foil, aluminum cans, antiperspirants, and some toothpastes. (See the recipes for homemade Lemongrass Natural Deodorant [page 259] and Toothpaste [page 260].)

Copper Cookware looks beautiful hanging in your kitchen and is an excellent conductor of heat; however, I do not recommend cooking with it. Uncoated copper can leach into your food, and even protective coatings will break down over time. Quality copper cookware is usually lined with tin, which can also wear off. Too much copper can suppress your zinc levels, weaken your immune system, and interfere with adrenal and thyroid function, which most commonly results in fatigue and exhaustion.

Small Appliances

Since antioxidant-packed smoothies and juices are essential to healing, it's important to choose the right tools. For smoothies, I recommend getting a high-powered blender. It turns whole fruits and vegetables into a smooth, full-bodied, satisfying smoothie. A juicer uses an extractor to separate the pulp and fiber from the juice, resulting in a light, refreshing beverage. (See Resources for brands.)

Blender Picking the right blender is essential to making rich and creamy smoothies. Many low-end blenders don't have the necessary pureeing power, and the motors sometimes burn out from the effort. When buying a blender for smoothies, buy the most powerful model you can afford. Generally, the higher-wattage models mean faster blade speeds without stressing the motor. You'll get better results. They tend to be more expensive, and as with most things, you get what you pay for. Also see which manufacturer has the best warranty.

Juicer There are two kinds of juicers: centrifugal and cold-press. The centrifugal juicer presses the fruit against a high-revolution-per-minute blade and relies on centrifugal force to send the juice out the spout while leaving the pulp behind. They work quickly and are less expensive than cold-press juicers, but it's sometimes difficult to juice leafy greens using one.

A cold-press juicer has blades that turn at a slower speed to preserve more of the fruit and vegetable nutrition and have no trouble with spinach, kale, and grasses. While costlier, you get more juice and nutrients from each piece of fruit or bunch of greens.

Electric Mixer From hand-held to standing mixers, these machines make fast work of repetitive cooking tasks like whisking together dry ingredients, pureeing root vegetables, and beating batters. Some models even have spiralizing and food processor attachments.

Food Processor This handy appliance comes in a wide range of sizes from mini to 14-cup models. The larger machines come with several blades that make short work of chopping and shredding vegetables, pureeing soups, and making batters and doughs. They are available at every price point. The mini models are ideal for chopping herbs, making pesto, or whipping up a salad dressing.

Instant Pot The newest appliance to make cooking less stressful is the Instant Pot. It's a time-saving electric appliance that consolidates a variety of cooking techniques—pressure cooking, slow cooking, sautéing, steaming, and keeping food warm. Since it has a pressure cooker setting, soups, stews, and other dishes can be ready in no time. This recently introduced handy countertop appliance speeds up cooking times and is energy efficient.

Slow Cooker This countertop appliance is best used for soups, stews, and braises, although you can use it for baking, puddings, and other dishes as well. Since food is cooked at low temperatures for long periods of time, the slow cooker is ideal for less-expensive, tougher cuts of meat like chuck roast, brisket, and lamb shanks.

Other Important Tools

Knives My dad was a great cook and taught me that good, sharp knives are the most important kitchen tools for cooks at every level. Quality, sharp knives make prepping food quicker and smoother. When shopping for knives, see how they feel when you grip the handle. The most basic ones to have in your kitchen are

- An all-purpose 8- to 10-inch chef's knife. It's the go-to knife for most food preparation, including slicing and dicing vegetables, meat, fish, and fruit.

- A 3½-inch paring knife. Use it for mincing garlic or slicing strawberries.

- A serrated knife with teeth. This is traditionally used for slicing bread, and it can also be used to slice citrus fruit and melons and foods with waxy surfaces, such as pineapples, watermelons, and citrus.

My dad also taught me to sharpen my knives regularly so they're always ready to use.

Mandoline You can use a knife to cut uniform, paper-thin slices of sweet potatoes, brussels sprouts, cucumbers, apples, onions, and other fruit and vegetables if you have good knife skills. For the rest of us, inexpensive mandolines can be found in housewares stores and online that make slicing fast and easy. Be sure to use the finger guards. You'll have a pile of evenly sliced vegetables in no time.

Parchment Paper Many of my recipes tell you to line a sheet pan with parchment paper. I recommend this for easy cleanup—once the food is cooked, discard the paper and give the pan a quick wipe. Look for untreated, chlorine-free parchment; parchment paper treated with chlorine is bright white in color, while unchlorinated, untreated parchment paper retains its natural brown color.

Spiralizer With this useful kitchen tool you can make fruit and vegetable "noodles" from apples and pears, summer and winter squash, beets, cucumbers, turnips, sweet potatoes, and more. You can cook the noodles or add them to salads and other dishes. Once the vegetable is secured in the spiralizer, you turn the handle and the blade produces precisely cut, thin noodles. Spiralizers range in price from $15 for the most basic version to hundreds of dollars for electric mixer attachments. You can also use a vegetable peeler, though the results will be more ribbonlike.

Sheet Pans These rectangular metal pans with rimmed edges on all four sides (cookie sheets have just two edges) are indispensable in my kitchen. I line them with parchment paper and use them to roast vegetables, fish, and chicken; to catch drips from baking sweet potatoes; and to bake cookies. Buy heavy, quality sheet pans—they often come packaged in multiples—so they will last for years. A full sheet pan measures 26 by 18 by ¾ inches, and a half sheet pan is 13 by 18 by ¾ inches. Both sizes will come in handy.

Meat Thermometer A meat thermometer guarantees that meat and poultry are cooked to a safe, but not underdone or overdone, temperature. Many of them are of poor quality and inaccurate. Invest in a quality meat thermometer, like the Super-Fast Thermapen. Don't take any chances. When cooking meat and poultry, use recommended guidelines on page 56. Remove the meat from the heat when it registers several degrees lower than the recommended temperature and let it rest. The temperature will rise as the meat rests (refer to cooking temperatures for meat on page 56).

Part Three

Nourishing You and Your Family

4

Breakfast

Start your day with exciting flavors, rich textures, and nourishing ingredients that will keep you full, focused, and energized until lunchtime! Say goodbye to sugar-laden cereals and inflammatory eggs as you feast your eyes and your taste buds on these sweet, savory, and satisfying breakfast dishes that will support your health from the very beginning of your day.

If you've been stuck in the "same old, same old" breakfast routine or are simply ready to enjoy exciting new options, these recipes will open your mind to a whole new world of breakfast ideas, as well as provide autoimmune-friendly recipes of classic family favorites.

Thanks to the popularity and availability of root-based flours such as cassava and tigernut, I am excited to include recipes for Sunday-morning favorites such as waffles, pancakes, biscuits, and muffins. As you enjoy these sweet and fluffy dishes, remember to pair them with a quality source of protein that will support your immune system and keep your blood sugar stable. If you think you have Candida overgrowth or SIBO (head to amymd.io/quiz to find out), please be sure to limit these until those infections have cleared.

In addition to these much-anticipated confections, you will notice a few of the all-time favorites from my books and website, such as Savory Breakfast Sausage (page 93) and Tigernut Oatmeal (page 98), along with many other dishes that will soon become tried-and-true go-to favorites in your kitchen!

BLC Tacos

As you can imagine, living in Texas and being married to a man whose last name is Garcia, making breakfast tacos is a must in our house! What are BLC Tacos? Bacon, lettuce, and chicken tacos: a few strips of bacon and some leftover chicken wrapped up in large lettuce leaves or Cassava Tortillas (page 100). A few sweet potato pieces and avocado complete this meal-in-a-hand.

1 sweet potato, peeled and chopped into ½-inch pieces

1 tablespoon avocado oil

4 slices pastured and nitrate-free bacon

¼ cup finely chopped onion

¼ teaspoon ground cinnamon

Fine sea salt and freshly ground black pepper, to taste

1 cup cooked and shredded chicken or leftover Herb Roasted Chicken (page 152)

4 large romaine lettuce leaves or 4 Cassava Tortillas (page 100)

½ avocado, sliced

Heat oven to 425°F. Place sweet potatoes on a sheet pan lined with parchment paper. Toss the potatoes with the avocado oil and bake for 30 minutes.

Put bacon in a cold skillet. Cook over medium-high heat for 3 minutes (or desired doneness), then turn bacon and cook to your liking. Remove bacon to paper towels to drain. Add onion and sweet potatoes to the skillet. Season with cinnamon, salt, and pepper. Cook until onion is softened. Add chicken to the pan to heat up.

Divide the mixture among lettuce leaves or tortillas and top with the avocado slices.

Turkey-Butternut Squash Hash

Serves 2

Hash is one of my go-to breakfasts and one of those recipes that you can play around with depending on what's in your fridge. No ground turkey? Some leftover cooked chicken or steak will do. Use cubes of sweet potato in place of squash, and spinach or swiss chard instead of kale. This hash, some Sweet Potato Biscuits (page 102), bowls of fresh berries, and cups of herbal tea make for the perfect weekend brunch.

1 tablespoon avocado oil

1 onion, chopped

1 garlic clove, minced

1 butternut squash, chopped

1 apple, cored and chopped

1 pound organic ground turkey

6 packed cups kale leaves

Fine sea salt and freshly ground black pepper, to taste

In a skillet, heat the avocado oil, onion, and garlic over medium heat. Sauté until the onion and garlic are soft.

Add the squash and apple. Cook, stirring occasionally, for 5 to 7 minutes or until the apples are cooked through and the squash is soft. Push to the side of the skillet. Add the turkey and cook until the meat has lost its pink color.

Stir in the kale, mix well, and cover. Cook for 5 minutes, or until the kale is wilted. Season with salt and pepper before serving.

Sweet Potato–Bacon Hash with Avocado Cream

Serves 2

In this hash, spices, cilantro, and avocado capture Southwestern flavors without using nightshade vegetables (tomatoes and peppers). It's a great way to use up leftover sweet potatoes, too.

2 sweet potatoes, peeled and cut into 1-inch cubes

2 tablespoons avocado oil

4 slices pastured and nitrate-free bacon

1 small red onion, diced

1 garlic clove, minced

1 teaspoon ground cumin

½ teaspoon ground coriander

½ teaspoon dried oregano

½ cup chopped cilantro leaves

Fine sea salt and freshly ground black pepper, to taste

1 avocado, pitted and peeled

1 lime, cut in wedges

Heat oven to 425°F. Place sweet potatoes on a sheet pan lined with parchment paper. Drizzle with avocado oil. Bake for 30 minutes.

While the sweet potatoes are roasting, put the bacon into a cold skillet, then turn on the heat to medium-high. Cook the bacon on both sides until crisp and transfer to a paper towel–lined plate. Add the onion, garlic, cumin, coriander, oregano, and half the cilantro to the skillet. Cook the onions until soft, about 5 minutes.

Add the sweet potatoes to the skillet. Season with salt and pepper. Cook, stirring occasionally, for 5 minutes.

In a bowl, mash the avocado. Add a squeeze of lime juice and combine.

Divide the hash between two plates and crumble the bacon over the top. Sprinkle on the remaining cilantro. Spoon on a dollop of mashed avocado and accompany with remaining lime wedges.

Spaghetti Squash Hash Browns

Makes 24 3-inch hash browns

The thinner the patties, the crisper they will be. Serve with Savory Breakfast Sausage (page 93) and sliced avocado. To smash the garlic, use the flat side of a chef's knife.

1 spaghetti squash, cut in half

2 garlic cloves, smashed into
    a paste

1 teaspoon freshly ground
    black pepper

½ teaspoon fine sea salt

1 tablespoon bacon fat

Heat oven to 450°F. Line a sheet pan with parchment paper.

Place the spaghetti squash cut-side down on the prepared pan. Bake for 45 minutes or until you can pierce the squash easily with a fork.

Remove from the oven, and when cool enough to handle, use a fork to scrape the "spaghetti" onto a clean towel. Squeeze out as much water as possible. Place the squash in a bowl; season with garlic, pepper, and salt. Use clean hands to mix well and blend in the garlic.

In a skillet, heat the bacon fat over medium-high heat. Divide the mixture into 24 round patties and cook until crisp, about 8 minutes on each side.

Roasted Sweet Potato Rounds with Smoked Salmon

Serves 2

Roasted sweet potato rounds, stand-ins for bagels, are topped with smoked salmon and avocado, then garnished with red onions and capers. Ideal for Sunday brunch or a first course at a dinner party. For a main course, arrange everything on a bed of salad greens with your choice of vinaigrette on the side.

1 sweet potato, peeled and cut into ¼-inch rounds

1 avocado, thinly sliced

1 4-ounce package sliced wild-caught smoked salmon

¼ red onion, thinly sliced

2 tablespoons capers, rinsed and drained

Heat oven to 350°F. Line a sheet pan with parchment paper.

Arrange the sweet potato slices on the prepared pan and bake for 10 minutes. Turn and bake the potatoes for another 10 minutes, or until soft when pierced with a knife. Once soft, place in a toaster oven to crisp up, about 5 minutes. As an option, you can cook the sweet potatoes in the toaster oven alone for 15 minutes, flipping halfway through.

Divide the sweet potatoes between two plates. Top each with avocado, smoked salmon, red onion, and capers.

Savory Breakfast Sausage

Makes 8 patties, serves 4

If you read The Autoimmune Solution, *then you know how amazing these breakfast sausage patties are and why I'm sharing the recipe again. I usually double or triple the recipe and freeze the extra patties so I have them quickly on hand for breakfast. Once the patties are cooked and cooled, wrap them individually in parchment paper and freeze for up to 1 month. Thaw overnight in the refrigerator and reheat in the oven or a skillet with a light brushing of avocado oil.*

Enjoy these patties at any meal. They also make a great snack when traveling. Enjoy with Wilted Greens with Bacon (page 193) and a spoonful or two of Spinach-Kale Pesto (page 196). I also include a sweeter variation with apples, cinnamon, and nutmeg.

1 pound free-range organic ground
   turkey or chicken

2 tablespoons finely chopped
   red onion

1 teaspoon minced garlic

¼ teaspoon fine sea salt

Pinch of ground mustard

Pinch of ground cumin

Pinch of freshly ground
   black pepper

1 tablespoon avocado oil

2 tablespoons Gut-Healing
   Bone Broth (page 71)
   or filtered water

In a large mixing bowl, combine the turkey, onion, garlic, salt, mustard, cumin, and pepper. Using clean hands, mix the meat and the seasonings together to incorporate the spices. Shape into eight patties.

Heat the avocado oil in a skillet over medium-high heat. Add the sausage patties and cook until brown, about 5 minutes on each side. Add the broth, cover the pan, and cook for 3 to 5 minutes.

Sweet Apple Breakfast Sausage: Omit the onion, garlic, mustard, cumin, and black pepper. To the ground turkey, add ½ teaspoon ground cinnamon, ¼ teaspoon ground nutmeg, ¼ teaspoon fine sea salt (as you would above), and ½ green apple, such as Granny Smith, finely chopped. Shape them into patties and then proceed as above.

Crunchy Maple Granola

Makes 2 cups

A huge jar of my mom's homemade granola could always be found in our kitchen. I was so disappointed when I learned that I couldn't eat granola because of my autoimmunity. Then tigernuts came along! Spoon a small amount of this granola onto your Coconut Milk Yogurt (page 70) or Acai Smoothie Bowl (page 99). A handful also makes a satisfying snack during the day. It's great to travel with as well.

½ cup sliced tigernuts

½ cup unsweetened coconut flakes

½ cup unsweetened shredded coconut

2 to 4 tablespoons maple syrup

1 teaspoon ground cinnamon

½ teaspoon ground nutmeg

¼ teaspoon fine sea salt

½ cup chopped dried cherries, cranberries, apples, or blueberries

Heat oven to 300°F. Line a sheet pan with parchment paper.

Combine all ingredients in a bowl and toss well. Spread the granola evenly on the prepared pan. Bake for 10 to 12 minutes, until the coconut is toasted. Watch to make sure that the coconut doesn't burn. Cool completely and store in a glass jar at room temperature.

Tigernut Waffles

Makes 2

If you thought that your waffle-making days were history, then I've got good news for you. Grain-free tigernut flour means you can once again have crisp, homemade waffles. The batter needs to be mixed in a food processor or blender to puree the plantain. If you're in the market for a new waffle iron, look for one that has a ceramic rather than a Teflon coating. For a sweet finish, drizzle a little maple syrup, raw honey, or one of the Fruit Compotes (page 211) on your waffles.

2 tablespoons coconut oil

¾ cup tigernut flour

¼ cup arrowroot flour

⅓ green plantain

½ teaspoon fine sea salt

½ teaspoon cream of tartar

¼ teaspoon baking soda

1 teaspoon ground cinnamon

1 tablespoon maple syrup

1 tablespoon pure vanilla extract

½ cup filtered water

Lightly oil a waffle iron with 1 tablespoon coconut oil, then heat according to the manufacturer's directions.

Combine all the ingredients and the remaining 1 tablespoon oil in a food processor or blender. Process until combined. While running the food processor, slowly pour in up to ½ cup water through the feed tube until the mixture forms the consistency of thick batter.

Pour about ½ cup batter onto the iron. Close the iron and cook until the waffle is done (it should be golden brown). When the first waffle is done, place on a warm platter and continue with the remaining batter.

Pumpkin Pancakes

Makes 4 4-inch pancakes

These pancakes are a weekend favorite of mine. Pumpkin is packed with beta-carotene, which is necessary for optimal immune and thyroid function. Be sure to buy canned pumpkin, rather than pumpkin pie filling.

2 tablespoons coconut oil

¼ cup tigernut flour

¾ cup arrowroot flour

2 tablespoons coconut flour

1 tablespoon The Myers Way Gelatin (or similar gelatin)

½ teaspoon fine sea salt

½ teaspoon cream of tartar

¼ teaspoon baking soda

1 tablespoon pumpkin pie spice

¼ cup canned pumpkin puree

2 tablespoons full-fat coconut milk

1 tablespoon pure maple syrup

1 tablespoon pure vanilla extract

In a skillet over medium heat, melt the coconut oil. Remove 1 tablespoon melted oil to a bowl.

Add the tigernut flour, arrowroot flour, coconut flour, gelatin, salt, cream of tartar, baking soda, and pie spice to a bowl and whisk together. Stir in the pumpkin puree, coconut milk, maple syrup, vanilla, and the remaining 1 tablespoon melted oil. Whisk together to make a thick batter.

Pour about ¼ cup batter into the skillet for each pancake. When bubbles appear on the pancakes and the sides start to firm up, turn and cook on the other side until golden brown.

Zucchini Muffins

Makes 12 muffins

These are my go-to baked goods when we have friends or family over for breakfast. Fragrant with cinnamon and nutmeg, these tasty muffins are great accompanied with Tigernut Butter (page 219) and a cup of herbal tea.

2 cups tigernut flour

½ cup cassava flour

2 teaspoons ground cinnamon

½ teaspoon ground nutmeg

1 teaspoon baking soda

1 teaspoon aluminum-free
   baking powder

1 tablespoon The Myers Way Gelatin
   (or similar gelatin)

2 ripe bananas, mashed

½ cup coconut oil

¼ cup honey

2 tablespoons freshly squeezed
   lemon juice

3 tablespoons filtered water

2 zucchinis, grated, with moisture
   squeezed out

Heat oven to 350°F. Line a muffin tin with twelve paper muffin cups.

In the bowl of a mixer, combine tigernut flour, cassava flour, cinnamon, nutmeg, baking soda, baking powder, and gelatin.

Add to the mixer bowl the mashed bananas, coconut oil, honey, lemon juice, and filtered water. Beat the ingredients together.

Using a spatula, gently fold in the grated zucchini. Divide the batter evenly among the muffin cups. Bake for 25 to 30 minutes, or until a toothpick comes out clean. Transfer the muffins to a rack and let cool.

Tigernut Oatmeal

Serves 2

Once again, amazing tigernuts to the rescue! Since most oatmeal is high in car-bohydrates and sugar, the added collagen and protein help balance blood sugar and provide more gut-healing benefits. Change up the toppings as desired.

1 cup sliced tigernuts

1 cup unsweetened shredded coconut

2 medium bananas, mashed

1 cup full-fat coconut milk

1 teaspoon ground cinnamon

1 scoop The Myers Way Collagen Protein (or similar collagen)

1 scoop The Myers Way Vanilla Paleo Protein (or similar protein powder)

1 cup filtered water

In a bowl, combine all ingredients. Cover and refrigerate overnight.

Place the mixture in a food processor or blender and pulse until mixture is the consistency of oatmeal. Enjoy the oatmeal chilled, or pour it into a saucepan and heat gently until hot.

Toppings

Berries and Cream: Stir in 1 cup mixed berries and 2 tablespoons coconut cream before refrigerating. Top with more coconut cream, if desired, before serving.

Tropical Tigernut Oats: Stir in ¼ cup pineapple before refrigerating.

Carrot Cake: Stir in ½ cup shredded carrot and 2 teaspoons maple syrup before refrigerating.

Acai Smoothie Bowl

Serves 2

Acai berries grow along the Amazon River in Brazil. They are loaded with antioxidants that can help build up your immune system and protect your cells against damage from free radicals. You can find Amafruits acai berry puree, organic and unsweetened, online and in many health food stores. Enjoy this smoothie bowl as is, or top it with unsweetened coconut flakes, banana slices, berries, Coconut Butter (page 69), Crunchy Maple Granola (page 94), pomegranate seeds, or sliced tigernuts.

4 4-ounce unsweetened frozen acai puree packets

1 banana, sliced

½ cup fresh blueberries

2 scoops The Myers Way Collagen Protein (or similar collagen)

½ cup full-fat coconut milk

Combine the acai, banana, blueberries, and collagen in a blender.

Through the opening in the blender's lid, slowly add coconut milk to desired consistency (you might not use all of the coconut milk). Sprinkle on toppings as desired.

Cassava Tortillas

Makes 8 4- to 5-inch tortillas

Being married to a man whose last name is Garcia, I had a hard time persuading my husband to give up his flour and corn tortillas until I discovered how to make them with cassava flour. They are so light and easily roll up just like other tortillas. You can fill cassava tortillas with roasted vegetables, crunchy salads, and grilled fish or chicken for tacos. A rolling pin is best for shaping and flattening the tortillas, or use a tortilla press, if you have one.

¾ cup cassava flour

2 tablespoons coconut flour

1 tablespoon coconut oil, melted

½ tablespoon apple cider vinegar

Pinch of fine sea salt

¾ cup filtered water

Arrowroot starch, for dusting

Put the cassava flour, coconut flour, oil, vinegar, salt, and water into a bowl. Stir well until a dough forms. Divide the dough into eight balls.

Place a sheet of parchment paper on a work surface and dust with the arrowroot starch to prevent sticking. Place one ball of dough on the floured parchment paper and place another sheet of parchment paper on top. Use a rolling pin to gently roll the ball into a 4- to 5-inch circle. Repeat with the remaining dough.

Heat a skillet over medium heat. Add a tortilla and cook about 3 minutes on each side. Repeat with the remaining tortillas.

Coconut Yogurt Parfaits

Serves 2

For a satisfying breakfast, afternoon snack, or dessert, layer Coconut Milk Yogurt (page 70), berries, and a bit of homemade granola in a glass. This recipe uses mixed berries, and you can layer your parfaits with whichever fruit is in season!

1 cup Coconut Milk Yogurt (page 70)

1 cup mixed fresh berries

1 cup Crunchy Maple Granola (page 94)

To make the parfaits, layer ¼ cup yogurt in a glass, followed by ¼ cup fruit, and ¼ cup granola. Repeat.

Sweet Potato Biscuits

Makes 12 biscuits

I come from the South, where everyone insists that his or her mom makes the best biscuits. If you like a more savory biscuit, mix 1 tablespoon chopped rosemary leaves into the batter. Sandwich a Savory Breakfast Sausage (page 93) between a split biscuit. While biscuits are always welcome on the breakfast table, you can also split them in half, fill with berries, and top with some Coconut Chocolate Mousse (page 245) for dessert.

1 to 2 sweet potatoes

½ cup full-fat coconut milk

¼ cup cassava flour

½ cup arrowroot flour

¼ cup coconut flour

1 tablespoon aluminum-free baking powder

1 teaspoon fine sea salt

⅓ cup palm shortening

Heat oven to 425°F. Pierce the sweet potatoes all over with a fork. Bake in oven for 45 minutes to 1 hour, until you can easily pierce the flesh with a knife. Once potatoes are cool enough to handle, slice open and scoop the flesh into a bowl and mash with a fork. Leave the oven on.

Line a sheet pan with parchment paper.

In a bowl, whisk together the mashed sweet potato and coconut milk. Add the cassava flour, arrowroot flour, coconut flour, baking powder, salt, and palm shortening and whisk well until all of the ingredients are combined.

Using a spoon or a cookie scoop, drop the batter onto the prepared sheet pan. Use the palm of your hand to gently press down on each biscuit to flatten. Bake for 14 to 16 minutes. Remove the biscuits to a rack to cool for a few minutes before serving.

Sweet Potato Biscuits with Savory
Breakfast Sausage, pages 102 and 93

Winter Salad with
Maple Vinaigrette,
page 145

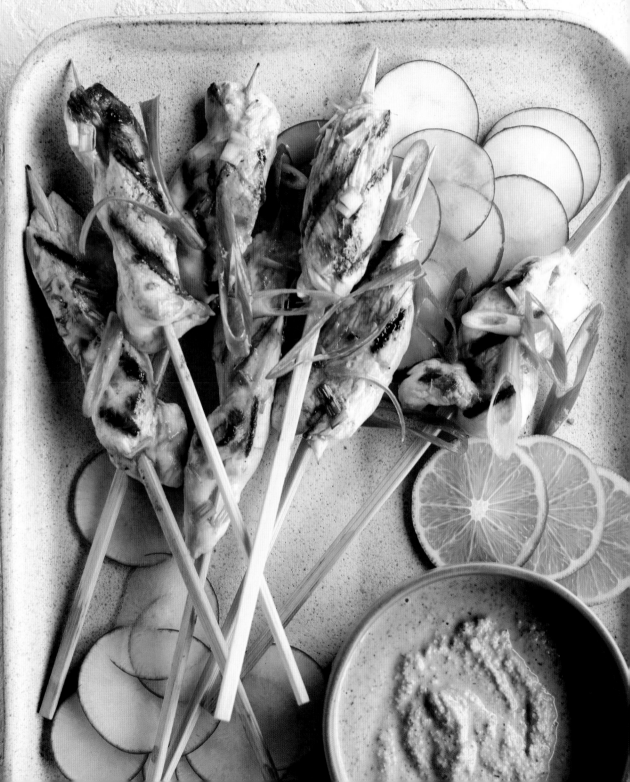

Chicken Satay with "Peanut" Sauce, pages 226 and 201

Butternut Squash–Sage Soup, page 138

Cucumber-Seaweed Salad, page 149

Creamy Zucchini-Basil Soup, page 136

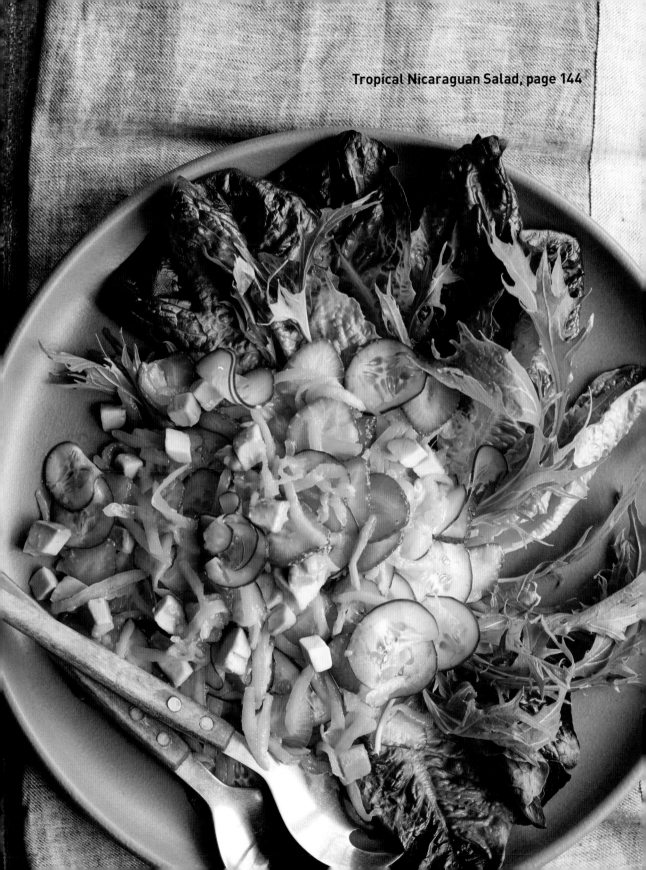

Tropical Nicaraguan Salad, page 144

Blackberry-Basil Mule, page 127

5

Smoothies,
Juices, and Other
Beverages

SMOOTHIES

Smoothies are my favorite way to get a delicious gut-healing, immune-supporting boost with virtually no effort. I keep big bags of fresh organic fruits and a superfoods greens mix in the freezer and The Myers Way Paleo Protein on my countertop so that I'm ready to make an energizing and satisfying smoothie at any time.

Smoothies are wonderful for anyone dealing with a leaky gut or poor digestion because the blending action breaks down the fruits and veggies so that they are easier for your body to digest and absorb. Adding The Myers Way Paleo Protein powder ensures that you're getting the essential amino acids you need in a form that your body can readily utilize. And don't forget, The Myers Way Collagen Protein upgrades any smoothie to a gut-healing and hair-, skin-, and nails-supporting powerhouse.

Here are my general guidelines for making a delicious, healing smoothie, and on the following pages you'll find my favorite flavorful combinations.

- 1 cup fruit, preferably berries

- 1 cup coarsely chopped vegetables (optional), such as leafy greens; cooked sweet potato, butternut squash, or pumpkin; summer squash

- ½ to 1 cup liquid, such as coconut milk, coconut water, or tigernut milk

- 1 tablespoon healthy fat, such as coconut, avocado, or flaxseed oil

- 1 scoop each The Myers Way Paleo Protein (or similar protein powder) and The Myers Way Collagen Protein (or similar collagen)

For each of the smoothies below, follow these instructions: Place all ingredients in a high-speed blender and blend until smooth. Here's a tip: Blend your smoothie twice. Turn the blender on for 20 seconds. Turn it off and let the contents settle. Blend again for another 20 seconds, and you'll have an extra smooth smoothie. Pour into a glass and enjoy!

Cherry Sunrise Smoothie

Serves 1

Cherries are loaded with antioxidants, making them an anti-inflammatory powerhouse. Fresh sweet cherries have a limited growing season, so when they are out of season, keep a bag of pitted organic frozen cherries on hand. Add them to juices and smoothies or toss a few in salads.

½ cup frozen pitted cherries
½ cup frozen mango cubes
½ cup full-fat coconut milk or
   filtered water
½ cup packed spinach
1 tablespoon coconut oil

1 scoop The Myers Way Vanilla
   Paleo Protein (or similar
   protein powder)
1 scoop The Myers Way Collagen
   Protein (or similar collagen),
   optional

Follow the instructions on page 104.

Very Berry Smoothie

Serves 1

If you're watching your blood sugar levels, believe it or not, steamed cauliflower is a healthy and creamy replacement for bananas in smoothies. I like to steam a big batch of it, let it cool, and throw it in the freezer to have on hand. Cauliflower is sugar free, and when it's steamed, it doesn't impart a sulfur-like flavor to your drink or affect your thyroid function. The vegetable has great hormone-balancing benefits, and both cauliflower and berries are packed with antioxidants, which play an important role in your immune system.

¼ cup frozen raspberries

¼ cup frozen blackberries

¼ cup frozen blueberries

½ cup cauliflower, steamed and then frozen

½ cup full-fat coconut milk

1 scoop The Myers Way Vanilla Paleo Protein (or similar protein powder)

1 scoop The Myers Way Collagen Protein (or similar protein powder), optional

Follow the instructions on page 104.

BANANAS FOR SMOOTHIES

Don't toss those overripe, dark-spotted bananas! Freeze and add them to smoothies for thicker texture and flavor. Peel the bananas. Cut them in half or into small pieces for easier blending. Arrange the banana pieces on a parchment-lined sheet pan and freeze. Once frozen, divide the equivalent of one or two bananas into individual containers that hold just enough for one or two smoothies.

Tropical Green Smoothie

Serves 1

I came up with this smoothie after a trip to Nicaragua. The fresh pineapple and mango take me back to the rushing ocean waves and white sandy beaches. The frozen avocado makes this smoothie so creamy—it's almost like ice cream. And the healthy fat from the avocado will keep you satisfied for hours.

½ cup frozen pineapple cubes

¼ cup frozen banana

¼ cup frozen mango cubes

1 cup packed fresh spinach leaves

½ cup unsweetened coconut water

¼ frozen avocado

1 scoop The Myers Way Vanilla Paleo Protein (or similar protein powder)

1 scoop The Myers Way Collagen Protein (or similar collagen), optional

Follow the instructions on page 104.

Mean Green Smoothie

Serves 1

This is a smoothie version of my favorite green juice. It's packed with B vitamins and healthy fats to support your immune system and adrenal glands.

½ cup spinach

¼ cup cubed cucumber

¼ frozen avocado

½ kiwi, peeled

¼ frozen banana (optional)

¼ cup filtered water

1 scoop The Myers Way Vanilla Paleo Protein (or similar protein powder)

1 scoop The Myers Way Collagen Protein (or similar collagen), optional

Follow the instructions on page 104.

Kale-Mint-Lemongrass Smoothie

Serves 1

This smoothie combines two of my favorite herbs—lemongrass and mint—to make a light and refreshing smoothie.

½ cup coconut milk

¼ frozen banana

1 cup baby kale leaves

3 mint leaves

½-inch piece lemongrass from the lower part of the stalk

1 scoop The Myers Way Vanilla Paleo Protein (or similar protein powder)

1 scoop The Myers Way Collagen Protein (or similar collagen), optional

Follow the instructions on page 104.

Dark Chocolate–Cherry Smoothie

Serves 1

If you crave chocolate-covered cherries, you will love this rich and decadent smoothie.

½ cup full-fat coconut milk

¾ cup frozen cherries

1 scoop The Myers Way Chocolate Paleo Protein (or similar protein powder)

¼ teaspoon ground cinnamon

1 scoop The Myers Way Collagen Protein (or similar collagen), optional

Follow the instructions on page 104.

Chai Smoothie

Serves 1

While traveling in India, I fell in love with chai tea. The tea and this smoothie are loaded with inflammation-fighting spices and all the warming and soothing flavors of a chai latte.

1 cup full-fat coconut milk

½ frozen banana

1 scoop The Myers Way Vanilla Paleo Protein (or similar protein powder)

1 scoop The Myers Way Collagen Protein (or similar collagen), optional

½ teaspoon ground cinnamon

½ teaspoon ground cardamom

½ teaspoon grated or minced ginger

½ teaspoon ground turmeric

¼ teaspoon ground nutmeg

¼ teaspoon ground cloves

Follow the instructions on page 104.

Strawberry Cheesecake Smoothie

Serves 1

Missing cheesecake? Well not anymore! This rich, dessert-like smoothie tastes just like the real thing without the inflammatory dairy and sugar. It's so filled with immune-supporting proteins and fats that it will keep you satisfied from breakfast to lunch.

1 cup frozen strawberries

½ cup full-fat coconut milk

1 tablespoon coconut butter

1 scoop The Myers Way Vanilla Paleo Protein (or similar protein powder)

1 scoop The Myers Way Collagen Protein (or similar collagen), optional

Follow the instructions on page 104.

Mint-Chocolate Chip Smoothie

Serves 1

Not just for breakfast, this ice cream–like smoothie is so rich and delicious that you could serve smaller portions for dessert. The spinach adds a boost of iron, vitamin B, and antioxidants. If you use mint leaves instead of essential oil, the smoothie will taste more citrusy than minty.

1 cup spinach leaves

1 drop peppermint essential oil or
    3 to 4 large mint leaves

½ cup full-fat coconut milk

1 to 2 tablespoons cacao nibs

1 scoop The Myers Way Vanilla
    Paleo Protein (or similar
    protein powder)

1 scoop The Myers Way Collagen
    Protein (or similar collagen),
    optional

½ frozen banana

Follow the instructions on page 104.

Gingerbread Cookie Smoothie

This smoothie takes me back to my childhood and reminds me of my mom. It tastes like a gingerbread cookie with all the flavors of my childhood and Christmas in a glass. Great for breakfast, dessert, or in place of eggnog at a holiday party.

½ cup full-fat coconut milk

¼ frozen banana

¼ teaspoon ground nutmeg

½ teaspoon ground cinnamon

¼ teaspoon ground ginger

⅛ teaspoon ground cloves

½ tablespoon molasses

1 scoop The Myers Way Vanilla Paleo Protein (or similar protein powder)

1 scoop The Myers Way Collagen Protein (or similar collagen), optional

Follow the instructions on page 104.

Pumpkin Pie Smoothie

Serves 1

Ditch that chemical- and sugar-laden pumpkin spice latte and opt for this instead! Here's another smoothie that can go from breakfast to dessert.

½ cup full-fat coconut milk

½ frozen banana

1 scoop The Myers Way Vanilla
   Paleo Protein (or similar
   protein powder)

1 scoop The Myers Way Collagen
   Protein (or similar collagen),
   optional

¼ cup canned pumpkin puree

½ teaspoon pumpkin pie spice

⅛ teaspoon ground ginger

Follow the instructions on page 104.

JUICES

Juices are a wonderful way to add to your diet more of the essential vitamins and minerals found in fruits and vegetables, while also enjoying a refreshing drink. If you love starting off your day with fresh juice, I recommend prepping your fruits and vegetables the night before so you'll have smooth sailing in the morning. Peel kiwis, citrus fruit (and also remove the bitter pith), and any other fruits and vegetables with skins that will affect the texture or taste of your juice.

Remember that you can always add The Myers Way Collagen Protein to any juice. Simply stir it in as soon as your juice is ready; it dissolves instantly and is tasteless. Collagen gives your juice a gut-healing boost and also adds protein to help balance the natural sugar of fruits.

As soon as your juice is ready, enjoy it right away so it doesn't separate or lose any of its nutritional value through oxidation. And here's a tip from my own experience: clean your juicer right after you use it for the easiest cleanup and so that it's ready to go the next time you're craving an energizing juice.

For each of the juices below, follow these instructions: With the motor of a juicer running, place each of the ingredients into the chute one at a time. For best results, use the food pusher to slowly push each of the ingredients down the chute. Juice will flow into the container, while the pulp will go into the pulp receptacle.

Splash of Sunshine

Serves 1

Packed with immune-supporting beta-carotene, energy-boosting B vitamins, and anti-inflammatory ginger, this juice is a great replacement for store-bought orange juice. Even on a rainy day, it's like drinking liquid sunshine.

¼ pineapple, peeled, cored, and chopped

2 orange carrots

1 sweet potato, chopped

1-inch piece of fresh ginger

Follow the instructions on page 114.

Purple Perfection

Serves 1

Filled with special antioxidants called carotenoids (such as lutein and zeaxanthin), flavonoids (such as rutin, resveratrol, and quercetin), and other antioxidant compounds like vitamins A, C, E, selenium, zinc, and phosphorus, this juice is sure to support your immune system. Kids will love both the purple color and the taste.

7 purple carrots

¼ cup blueberries

1 apple, cored and chopped

¼ cucumber

½ beet

½ lemon

Follow the instructions on page 114.

Classic Detoxifying Green Juice

Serves 1

This juice is an all-around immune booster and detoxifier in a glass. Chlorophyll, the green pigment found in plants, has been shown to increase red blood cell count and calm inflammation. Cilantro helps tame the toxins by binding heavy metals and supporting detoxification. Lemon helps flush the lymphatic system. And bioactive substances in ginger help to reduce inflammation and infections.

1 handful kale and/or spinach
   leaves
1 cucumber
1 pear, cored and chopped

4 celery stalks
1 lemon, peeled
¼-inch piece of fresh ginger
Handful of cilantro

Follow the instructions on page 114.

Free-Radical Fighter

Serves 1

Free radicals overwhelm our bodies and can lead to early aging. Fruits and vegetables rich in antioxidants, like the ones in this juice, are our best defense. Drink it in the afternoon for a refreshing free-radical flush.

2 apples, cored and chopped

1 cucumber

1 cup blueberries

2 cups red or purple grapes

1 cup spinach

1-inch piece of fresh ginger

Follow the instructions on page 114.

Organic Green Margarita Juice

Serves 1

I often start my day off with this juice, flushing out the night's toxins with the cilantro. It's great as a refresher after a workout, too. Or serve it in shot glasses with appetizers at a Mexican-themed dinner.

1½ packed cups baby spinach

1 lime

1 gala apple

1 cucumber

1 cup cilantro

Follow the instructions on page 114.

OTHER BEVERAGES

Smoothies and juices aren't the only delicious beverages that can support your health. From inflammation-fighting Golden Milk (page 120) to fizzy fruit mocktails, there are lots of creative drink ideas for every season.

To give a gut-repairing boost to any of these delicious drinks, while supporting beautiful hair skin, and nails, simply add one scoop of The Myers Way Collagen Protein or an easy upgrade.

And whether you're snuggling under a warm comforter with an autoimmune-friendly Pumpkin Spice Latte (page 122) or enjoying a Blackberry-Basil Mule (page 127) by the pool, remember to relax and relish the moment—after all, Relieve Your Stress is part of the fourth pillar of The Myers Way.

Golden Milk

Serves 2

The turmeric in this warming drink gives it a sunshine golden color, while turmeric's active ingredient, curcumin, is a potent antioxidant praised for reducing the inflammation and pain of autoimmunity and other chronic health conditions. Curcumin is absorbed best when consumed with some fat from the coconut oil and black pepper.

2 cups unsweetened coconut milk

1-inch piece of turmeric, sliced

1 cinnamon stick

½-inch piece of fresh ginger, sliced

Dash of freshly ground black pepper

1 scoop The Myers Way Collagen Protein (or similar collagen)

2 tablespoons coconut oil

Bring coconut milk to a simmer on the stove with the turmeric, cinnamon stick, ginger, and black pepper, and then simmer for about 10 minutes. Once warm, strain coconut milk and pour into blender or food processor. Add the collagen (if desired) and coconut oil and blend until frothy.

Peppermint Hot Chocolate

Serves 2

Unsweetened cocoa powder is packed with nutrients including iron, manganese, magnesium, and zinc. Iron and zinc are essential to maintaining optimal immune function. The flavonoids in cocoa function as antioxidants that help prevent systemic inflammation. This beverage is smooth and creamy, with a minty flavor, and will warm you up on a chilly night.

3 tablespoons unsweetened cocoa powder

3 tablespoons filtered water

1 can full-fat coconut milk

1 drop peppermint essential oil

In a bowl, combine cocoa powder and water. Set aside. Pour the coconut milk into a saucepan and bring to a boil; then remove from heat. Let cool for 1 or 2 minutes, then pour into a high-speed blender. Add the cocoa powder mixture and peppermint oil. Blend until frothy, about 20 seconds. Serve immediately.

Pumpkin Spice Latte (Upgraded)

Serves 2

Ditch that chemical- and sugar-laden pumpkin spice latte from your local coffee shop and opt for this healthier option instead! If you have pumpkin pie spice in your spice drawer, use 2 teaspoons of that in place of the cinnamon, ginger, nutmeg, and clove below. This upgraded version includes The Myers Way Collagen Protein for an extra boost of gut-repairing properties.

½ cup pumpkin puree

1 teaspoon ground cinnamon

½ teaspoon ground ginger

½ teaspoon ground nutmeg

½ teaspoon ground clove

2 tablespoons maple syrup or
   coconut sugar

2 cups full-fat coconut milk

2 tablespoons pure vanilla extract

1 scoop The Myers Way Collagen
   Protein (or similar collagen)

In a saucepan over medium heat, combine pumpkin puree, spices, and maple syrup or coconut sugar. Stir and heat for 2 minutes until fragrant. Add the coconut milk and vanilla. Bring to a simmer. Pour into a food processor and blend until frothy, about 20 seconds. Pour into two cups and serve.

Chai Tea Latte (Upgraded)

Serves 2

This latte is loaded with inflammation-fighting spices and warming and soothing flavors. The dandelion root tea in the ingredients doesn't contain any caffeine and tastes just like coffee. Look for "roasted" dandelion root, which is more flavorful. This upgraded version includes The Myers Way Collagen Protein for an extra boost of gut-repairing properties.

8 cardamom seeds

8 cloves

4 black peppercorns

2 whole cinnamon sticks

1-inch piece of ginger, peeled

2 cups coconut milk

2 pitted dates, chopped

2 cups filtered water

2 scoops The Myers Way Collagen Protein (or similar collagen)

4 roasted dandelion root tea bags

Place all ingredients except collagen and tea bags in a saucepan and bring to a boil; then lower the heat to a simmer and cook for 10 minutes. Remove from heat.

Whisk in the collagen and add the tea bags. Steep for another 10 minutes.

Strain the latte into two cups.

French Vanilla Coffee Creamer

Makes 16 tablespoons

This creamer is a great replacement for classic store-bought coffee creamers, which tend to be high in sugar and other unnecessary ingredients, even if they don't have any dairy. If you want a richer vanilla taste, try adding fresh vanilla bean instead of using extract.

1 cup full-fat coconut milk

1 scoop The Myers Way Collagen Protein (or similar collagen)

⅛ teaspoon stevia

1 teaspoon pure vanilla extract

In a saucepan, bring coconut milk to a boil and then remove from heat.

Whisk in collagen, stevia, and vanilla extract.

Pour into a glass storage container and let cool, stirring occasionally to prevent the creamer from solidifying.

Store in refrigerator.

Creamy Hot Chocolate

Serves 2

When making hot chocolate, be sure to use pure unsweetened cocoa powder rather than sugary, processed cocoa mixes. The Myers Way Paleo Protein adds a nutritional boost to a warming favorite.

2 cups full-fat coconut milk

2 scoops The Myers Way Chocolate Paleo Protein Powder (or similar protein powder)

½ teaspoon ground cinnamon

In a saucepan, bring coconut milk to a boil and then remove from heat.

Whisk in the protein powder and cinnamon and pour into mugs.

Gut-Soothing Collagen Tea

Serves 2

If you don't have time to make Gut-Healing Bone Broth (page 71), this collagen tea is a super quick alternative. It does everything from helping to repair a leaky gut; supporting strong hair, skin, and nails; and improving liver function. Flavorless and colorless collagen silently does its job when stirred into a cup of tea. The ginger fights inflammation, and the lemon detoxifies.

2 cups filtered water

½-inch piece of ginger, peeled and cut in half

1 tablespoon lemon juice

2 scoops The Myers Way Collagen Protein (or similar collagen)

Bring the water to a boil, and then remove from heat.

Put a piece of ginger and half the lemon juice in two tea cups. Pour hot water into the cups and let steep for 10 minutes.

Stir 1 scoop collagen into each cup before drinking.

Blackberry-Basil Mule

Serves 2

This "mocktail" is a fun and delicious twist on the classic Moscow mule. Some beverage recipes call for "muddling" herbs and fruit. To muddle, put the ingredients in a sturdy glass and use the end of a wooden spoon or a muddler and press down on whatever the recipe calls for to release essential oils and juices.

1 cup sliced ginger

½ cup coconut sugar

¾ cup filtered water

1 cup blackberries

3 fresh basil leaves, chopped

1 lime

1 cup sparkling water

To make ginger concentrate, add the ginger, coconut sugar, and water to a saucepan. Bring to a boil; then lower the heat and simmer for 10 minutes. Remove from heat and let cool for 1 hour. Strain out the ginger.

Divide blackberries and basil between two glasses. Muddle into the bottom. Squeeze ½ lime into each glass. Add 3 tablespoons ginger concentrate to each glass, then add ½ cup sparkling water to each and mix to combine.

Strawberry Mojito

Serves 2

Mint is so easy to grow whether you have a small pot on a balcony or a full garden. What to do with all that fresh mint? Make strawberry mojitos! Serve with Five-Vegetable Guacamole (page 220) and Cassava Tortillas (page 100).

20 fresh mint leaves

10 fresh strawberries, tops removed

Juice of 1 lime

2 teaspoons coconut sugar (optional)

1 cup sparkling water

Divide mint leaves and strawberries into two glasses.

Muddle together in the glass. If desired, add ice to glasses.

Divide remaining ingredients into each glass, stir, and serve.

Rosemary-Lemon Spritzer

Serves 2

Rosemary is very easy to grow and does not need a lot of space. We have a large bush outside our front door. In the summer, I often double or triple the rosemary-lemon concentrate and keep a jar in the refrigerator to make these quick, refreshing mocktails.

1 cup freshly squeezed lemon juice

1 sprig fresh rosemary

⅛ teaspoon stevia (optional)

2 cups sparkling water

In a saucepan, bring lemon juice, rosemary, and stevia to a boil; then lower the heat to a simmer and cook for 3 minutes.

Transfer to a storage container and let cool in refrigerator for 1 hour.

Strain mixture.

Pour 1 cup sparkling water into each glass. Then add 6 tablespoons rosemary-lemon concentrate to each glass and serve.

Sangria

Serves 2

My version of this classic Spanish punch has just the right hint of sweetness without the hangover. Enjoy it on a hot summer's night with a Chicken Burrito Bowl (page 157) or Five-Vegetable Guacamole (page 220) and Cassava Tortillas (page 100).

½ apple, chopped

½ pear, chopped

1 cup unsweetened cranberry-grape juice

2 tablespoons freshly squeezed lemon juice

1 cup sparkling water

Combine apples, pears, cranberry-grape juice, and lemon juice in a glass jar.

Cover and shake.

Let sit for 1 hour or overnight.

Shake before using and divide between two glasses.

Top each with ½ cup sparkling water and stir.

Agua Fresca

Serves 4

This is my go-to weekend drink on hot Texas summer days. It's light, sweet, and refreshing—and another great way to use fresh mint.

3 cups watermelon or fruit of choice

1½ cups sparkling water

Juice from 1 lemon

16 mint leaves

Puree watermelon in blender or food processor. Strain out the pulp using a fine sieve, or use as is with the pulp.

In your favorite summertime pitcher, mix melon puree, sparkling water, and lemon. Pour into glasses and garnish with mint leaves.

6

Soups and Salads

Soups are among my favorite gut-healing and immune-supporting foods. A cup of Gut-Healing Bone Broth (page 71) in the morning or evening is soothing, nourishing, and best of all, easy to make! In the winter, our dinner favorites are Curried Carrot Soup (page 137) and Roasted Vegetable Soup (page 139), and I am constantly finding creative new ways to enjoy the healing properties of comforting soups. I've adapted a variety of styles from around the world—Mexican tortilla soup, Thai meatball soup, and creamy chowder to share with you.

And I've gotten even more creative when it comes to salads, thanks to a lifetime of enjoying their delicious crunch and bright flavors. In fact, when I was growing up, my family had a salad on the table every night, and I have continued that tradition with my own family. I love seeing dark leafy greens on my table, such as spinach, baby kale, arugula, or watercress and knowing we are about to enjoy a delicious dose of immune-supporting vitamin A, folate, and B vitamins.

There are so many options and combinations when it comes to salads that there's always something new to try! For instance, try cutting your vegetables into different shapes or use a spiralizer to make long ribbons of zucchini or carrots.

Chicken "Noodle" Soup

Serves 2

Modernized and upgraded, this classic soup includes immune-supporting ginger, turmeric, and Gut-Healing Bone Broth (page 71). Spiralized zucchini acts as the noodles.

1 tablespoon avocado oil

½ onion, chopped

1 clove garlic, minced

3 carrots, chopped

2 stalks celery, chopped

1 teaspoon grated fresh ginger

4 cups Gut-Healing Bone Broth (page 71)

1½ tablespoons grated fresh turmeric

1 cup cooked and shredded chicken or leftover Herb Roasted Chicken (page 152)

1 zucchini, spiralized or julienned

In a large saucepan or Dutch oven, heat the oil, onion, and garlic over medium heat and sauté for 1 minute. Add the carrots, celery, and ginger. Sauté the vegetables until soft.

Add the bone broth and turmeric. Bring to a boil, lower the heat, and simmer for 5 minutes.

Stir in the chicken and zucchini and cook for another 3 minutes to heat through. Divide between two bowls and serve.

Chicken Tortilla Soup

Serves 2

This is a healthier version of the Southwest classic. A squeeze of lime adds brightness, Cassava Tortilla chips offer some crunch, and cilantro adds a hint of citrusy taste to this soup.

½ pound free-range chicken or leftover Herb Roasted Chicken (page 152)

2 Cassava Tortillas (page 100)

1 tablespoon avocado oil

½ onion, chopped

2 cloves garlic, minced

4 carrots, chopped

4 cups Gut-Healing Bone Broth (page 71)

½ cup cilantro leaves, plus additional for garnish

Juice of ½ lime

1 avocado, diced

Heat oven to 400°F. Cook chicken for 18 to 20 minutes or until cooked through. Set aside. Once cool enough to handle, shred chicken.

Slice Cassava Tortillas into triangles or strips. Place on a parchment-lined baking sheet and bake for 10 to 15 minutes, until tortillas have crisped up like chips.

In a large saucepan, heat avocado oil, onion, and garlic. Sauté for 2 to 3 minutes. Add carrots and sauté another 3 minutes. Add the bone broth and chicken. Bring to a boil, then reduce heat to a simmer and cook for 10 minutes.

Add cilantro, lime, and avocado to saucepan and stir together. Ladle into bowls and serve with tortilla chips.

Creamy Zucchini-Basil Soup

Serves 2

Zucchini is rich in vitamin A, zinc, folate, and other B vitamins that are essential to optimal thyroid and immune function. This recipe is rich and creamy. Double or triple the recipe to serve as a starter for a party.

1 tablespoon avocado oil

1 onion, finely chopped

2 zucchinis, chopped

2 cups Gut-Healing Bone Broth
  (page 71)

¼ cup basil leaves

1 clove garlic, minced

Fine sea salt and freshly ground
  black pepper, to taste

¼ cup extra virgin olive oil

In a saucepan, heat the oil and onion over medium-high heat. When hot, add the zucchini and sauté until the vegetables are soft. Set aside and let cool for 5 minutes.

Place the zucchini and onion, bone broth, basil, garlic, salt, and pepper in a food processor. Blend until combined. Add the olive oil and pulse until combined.

Return the soup to the saucepan and reheat. Divide soup between two bowls and serve.

Curried Carrot Soup

Serves 2

This soup is filled with beta-carotene and vitamin A for optimal immune and thyroid function as well as turmeric, ginger, and bone broth to prevent inflammation and heal your gut. Good stand-ins for the carrots are an equal amount of sweet potatoes, parsnips, butternut squash, or cauliflower or a combination of two or three vegetables. Follow the soup with grilled fish and Mango-Avocado Salsa (page 210).

1 tablespoon avocado oil

6 carrots, chopped

½ onion, chopped

1 teaspoon grated fresh ginger

1½ cups Gut-Healing Bone Broth (page 71)

1 teaspoon ground cumin

½ teaspoon ground turmeric

½ teaspoon ground black pepper

¼ teaspoon fine sea salt

1 cup full-fat coconut milk (or coconut cream for thicker consistency)

Juice from ¼ lime

½ cup chopped cilantro leaves, for garnish

In a large saucepan, combine avocado oil, carrots, onion, and ginger over medium heat. Sauté until soft.

Stir in the bone broth, cumin, turmeric, pepper, and salt. Bring soup to a boil; then reduce heat to a simmer and cook for 10 minutes. Remove from heat and allow the soup to cool slightly.

Puree the soup in a food processor or blender. Then return it to the saucepan and stir in coconut milk and lime juice. Simmer over low heat just until hot.

Divide the soup between two bowls and garnish with chopped cilantro.

Butternut Squash–Sage Soup

Serves 2

Butternut squash is one of my favorite winter vegetables. It's packed with beta-carotene and vitamin A for immune support and is also very satisfying. The rosemary and sage offer a savory flavor, and the garlic and bacon will have your family or friends asking for more. When roasting the vegetables, add one or two halved and seeded apples to the sheet pan for a sweet touch.

½ butternut squash, peeled and chopped

½ onion, chopped

1 clove garlic, whole

3 fresh sage leaves

1 sprig fresh rosemary

2 slices pastured and nitrate-free bacon, chopped

2 cups Gut-Healing Bone Broth (page 71)

Fine sea salt and freshly ground black pepper, to taste

2 tablespoons full-fat coconut milk

Heat oven to 450°F. Line a sheet pan with parchment paper.

Arrange the butternut squash, onion, garlic clove, sage, and rosemary on the sheet pan. Roast for 30 minutes or until butternut squash can be pierced with a fork.

While the vegetables are roasting, cook the bacon in a saucepan until crisp. Drain on a paper towel–lined plate. Chop into small pieces. Reserve the bacon fat for another use.

Remove the vegetables from the oven and let cool for 10 minutes. Place the vegetables, broth, salt, and pepper in a food processor and puree. Pour the soup into a saucepan and bring to a boil. Reduce the heat and stir in the coconut milk. Divide the soup between two bowls and garnish with the bacon pieces.

Roasted Vegetable Soup

Serves 4

Cruciferous vegetables such as brussels sprouts and broccoli are some of the most nutrient-dense foods on the planet. They are fully cooked in this soup, so those people with thyroid dysfunction can enjoy abundant amounts of this soup. The garlic and shallots are sulfur-rich compounds that help to make the most potent detoxifier in our bodies, glutathione. This soup is ideal for a winter's dinner followed by Winter Salad with Maple Vinaigrette (page 145).

1 pound brussels sprouts, halved

1 pound broccoli florets, chopped

2 tablespoons avocado oil

2 shallots, chopped

1 clove garlic, minced

3 cups Gut-Healing Bone Broth
   (page 71)

¼ cup full-fat coconut milk

½ teaspoon fine sea salt

Freshly ground black pepper,
   to taste

Heat oven to 425°F. Line a sheet pan with parchment paper. Arrange brussels sprouts and broccoli on the pan in a single layer and drizzle with 1 tablespoon avocado oil. Roast for 25 to 30 minutes, turning halfway through, until the vegetables can be pierced with a fork.

While the vegetables are roasting, put 1 tablespoon oil, shallots, and garlic in a skillet over medium-high heat and sauté for 2 to 3 minutes.

Remove brussels sprouts and broccoli from oven and let cool for 5 to 10 minutes. Reserve ½ cup of each vegetable. Add the remaining vegetables, shallots, garlic, bone broth, coconut milk, salt, and pepper to a food processor and puree. Blend until combined. Pour the soup into a saucepan and reheat. Divide the soup among four bowls and garnish with the remaining roasted brussels sprouts and broccoli.

Cauliflower Chowder

Serves 4

*Cauliflower is a nutrient-dense cruciferous vegetable. The bacon adds smoki-
ness to this thick, creamy soup. Rich and filling, it will be a cold weather favorite.*

4 slices pastured and
   nitrate-free bacon

1 carrot, coarsely chopped

1 stalk celery, coarsely chopped

1 clove garlic, minced

½ head cauliflower, coarsely
   chopped

1 bay leaf

1 cup full-fat coconut milk

2 cups Gut-Healing Bone Broth
   (page 71)

½ teaspoon fine sea salt

½ 15-ounce can coconut cream

In a Dutch oven, cook the bacon until crisp over medium-high heat. Drain the
bacon on paper towels and crumble. Reserve the bacon fat.

Add the carrots, celery, and garlic to the bacon fat. Sauté for 3 to 5 minutes,
until softened. Add the cauliflower and sauté 5 minutes. Add the bay leaf,
coconut milk, bone broth, and salt. Bring to a boil, and then lower the heat and
simmer for 10 minutes or until cauliflower is fork tender. Remove soup from
the heat and allow it to cool slightly. Remove the bay leaf.

Put half the soup in a food processor and puree. Return to the pot with the
remaining soup. Stir in the coconut cream and reheat. Divide the soup among
four bowls and top with the bacon.

Thai Meatball Soup

Serves 4

Ginger and fish sauce impart authentic flavors to this Thai-inspired popular street food favorite. Big bowls of broth and vegetables make this a complete meal.

Meatballs

- 1 pound ground organic turkey
- 2 tablespoons coconut aminos
- 1 tablespoon chopped cilantro
- ½ tablespoon grated fresh ginger
- 1 teaspoon fish sauce
- 2 green onions, chopped

Broth

- 8 cups Gut-Healing Bone Broth (page 71)
- 3 carrots, shredded
- 1 zucchini, shredded
- 1 yellow squash, shredded
- 2 green onions, chopped
- 2 tablespoons coconut aminos
- 1 tablespoon toasted sesame oil
- 1 tablespoon grated fresh ginger
- ½ teaspoon fish sauce
- Juice of 1 lime
- ¼ cup chopped cilantro, for garnish

To make the meatballs: Heat oven to 375°F. Line a sheet pan with parchment paper.

In a bowl, combine turkey, coconut aminos, cilantro, ginger, fish sauce, and green onion. Using clean hands, mix and shape the mixture into 1-inch meatballs. Arrange meatballs on the prepared pan and bake for 30 minutes.

To make the broth: Put the bone broth, carrots, zucchini, squash, green onions, coconut aminos, sesame oil, ginger, fish sauce, and lime juice into a Dutch oven. Bring to a boil; then lower the heat and simmer until the vegetables are cooked through. Add the cooked meatballs to the soup and simmer for 1 to 2 minutes. Divide among four bowls and garnish with chopped cilantro.

Brussels Sprouts and Red Cabbage Salad

Serves 4

Make this colorful, crunchy winter salad when garden-fresh lettuces and other greens aren't available. Shaving the sprouts and shredding the cabbage using a mandoline will save time. Be careful not to overdo this salad if you have thyroid dysfunction.

3 cups shredded brussels sprouts

1 cup shredded red cabbage

1 apple, cored and diced

¼ cup dried cranberries

2 tablespoons extra virgin olive oil

2 tablespoons apple cider vinegar

1 tablespoon maple syrup

1 teaspoon organic Dijon mustard

1 tablespoon avocado oil

2 shallots, thinly sliced, for garnish

In a bowl, combine the brussels sprouts, cabbage, apple, and cranberries.

In a separate bowl, whisk together the olive oil, vinegar, maple syrup, and mustard. Toss the dressing with the salad to coat evenly.

Heat the avocado oil in a skillet over medium-high heat. Add the shallots and cook until crispy, taking care so they don't burn. Sprinkle the shallots over the salad.

Mardi Gras Salad

Serves 4

*My grandmother lived right on the Mardi Gras parade route in New Orleans,
which meant our family hosted a party almost every night during the season. A
Mardi Gras salad is anything that contains Mardi Gras colors—purple, green,
and gold. The brussels sprouts, red cabbage, cauliflower, and butternut squash
in this adaptation of my grandmother's Mardi Gras salad caramelize beautifully
with high-temperature roasting. Tangy pomegranate seeds add a bit of sweetness.*

Salad

4 cups halved brussels sprouts

½ head red cabbage, chopped into
   1-inch pieces

½ butternut squash, chopped into
   1-inch pieces

1 head cauliflower, roughly chopped

3 tablespoons avocado oil

Fine sea salt, to taste

Freshly ground black pepper,
   to taste

1 cup pomegranate seeds

Dressing

½ tablespoon prepared
   horseradish

1 clove garlic, minced

½ shallot, minced

1 teaspoon honey

1 teaspoon apple cider vinegar

1 tablespoon Dijon mustard

¼ cup extra virgin olive oil

Heat oven to 400°F. Line two sheet pans with parchment paper.

To make the salad: Place the brussels sprouts and cabbage on one prepared
pan and the squash and cauliflower on the other prepared pan. Drizzle the
avocado oil over the vegetables, and using clean hands, toss to coat. Then
arrange the vegetables in a single layer. Season with the salt and pepper.
Roast the brussels sprouts and cabbage for 20 minutes and the butternut
squash and cauliflower for 40 minutes.

To make the dressing: While the vegetables are roasting, whisk together
dressing ingredients. Combine roasted vegetables in a large bowl. Toss with
the dressing and sprinkle with pomegranate seeds. Serve warm.

Tropical Nicaraguan Salad

Serves 2

At my first dinner while on vacation in Nicaragua, I ordered this salad. Fresh greens were topped with a rainbow of fruits and vegetables—mango, strawberries, cucumber, and avocado—and then drizzled with a simple dressing of olive oil and vinegar. I loved it so much that I ate it every day during my vacation, and I now frequently make it at home.

4 to 6 cups organic mixed
    field greens

¼ to ½ mango, peeled and grated

½ cup strawberries, thinly sliced

½ cucumber, thinly sliced

1 avocado, diced

¼ teaspoon fine sea salt

2 tablespoons extra virgin olive oil

2 teaspoons apple cider vinegar

In a large salad bowl combine greens, mango, strawberries, cucumber, and avocado.

In a small bowl mix together salt, oil, and vinegar.

Drizzle desired amount of dressing over salad and serve.

AVOCADOS

Avocados contain twenty vitamins and thirteen essential minerals. Their potassium content is three times that of a banana, and they're high in fiber. It's no wonder that this was the first food I fed to Elle when she turned six months old. The pebbly organic Hass avocados from California taste better and have more good-for-you monounsaturated fat and less water than the smooth-skinned Florida variety. We eat two avocados a day in our house. To speed ripening, seal avocados in a brown paper bag for a day or two. You can also freeze the fruit whole or cut it in half.

Winter Salad with Maple Vinaigrette

Makes 2 large salads or 4 side salads

Kale, arugula, and watercress are all nutrient-dense and vitamin-rich cruci-ferous greens that are flavorful and support your immune system. They are available throughout the year so you can make this salad even during the coldest months.

Salad
- ½ red onion, sliced
- ¼ cup apple cider vinegar
- ½ teaspoon salt
- 1 apple, thinly sliced
- 3 cups kale
- 3 cups arugula or watercress

Dressing
- ½ cup extra virgin olive oil
- 4 tablespoons apple cider vinegar
- 3 tablespoons maple syrup
- ½ teaspoon fine sea salt
- ¼ teaspoon freshly ground black pepper

Combine onion, apple cider vinegar, and salt in glass storage container. Let sit for at least 2 hours.

When onions are ready, heat oven to 400°F. Place apple slices on a parchment paper–lined sheet pan and roast for 20 minutes.

While apples are roasting, whisk together dressing ingredients. Remove apples from oven. In a large bowl, toss together apples, kale, arugula, and red onions. Top salad with dressing and toss to coat.

Apricot-Chicken Salad

Serves 2

Apricots in this chicken salad add color and brighten its flavor. Apricots are also rich in beta-carotene and are excellent sources of cobalt, copper, and iron—important nutrients in maintaining a healthy gut.

1 celery stalk, chopped

½ cup dried apricots, chopped

¼ red onion, finely chopped

1 cup cooked and shredded chicken or leftover Herb Roasted Chicken (page 152)

2 tablespoons Aïoli (page 197)

½ tablespoon Dijon mustard

¼ teaspoon freshly ground black pepper

Combine all ingredients in a bowl and mix together. Serve over lettuce or with Rosemary–Sea Salt Crackers (page 222).

Tangy Coleslaw

Serves 4

Being from the South, I couldn't write a cookbook without a coleslaw recipe. Coleslaw makes the perfect accompaniment to The Perfect Fast Man Burgers (page 162), Carolina Pulled Pork (page 169), or grilled fish. If you're having people over for a barbecue, double or triple the recipe.

2 cups shredded red cabbage

2 cups shredded green cabbage

2 cups shredded carrots

¼ cup extra virgin olive oil

3 tablespoons apple cider vinegar

1 tablespoon honey

2 cloves garlic, minced

½ teaspoon fine sea salt

½ teaspoon Dijon mustard

½ teaspoon celery seed

½ teaspoon freshly ground
black pepper

In a bowl, toss together the cabbages and carrots.

In a separate bowl, whisk together the olive oil, vinegar, honey, garlic, salt, mustard, celery seed, and pepper.

Pour the dressing over the vegetable mixture to coat thoroughly.

Store in refrigerator until ready to serve or for 3 to 4 days.

Herbed "Potato" Salad

Serves 2

Steamed white root vegetables stand in for the traditional white potatoes in this "potato" salad. A handful of fresh green herbs adds flavor and brightness. Serve as a side dish with The Perfect Fast Man Burgers (page 162), the World's Best Asian Flank Steak (page 161), or Braised Pork Ribs (page 171).

1 pound mixed white root vegetables (such as rutabagas, parsnips, white sweet potatoes, turnips), peeled and cut into bite-size pieces

3 tablespoons apple cider vinegar

3 tablespoons extra virgin olive oil

½ cup mixed chopped fresh herbs (such as parsley, dill, chives)

1 shallot, minced

Fine sea salt and freshly ground black pepper, to taste

Place a steamer basket in a large saucepan. Add 2 inches of water. Arrange the vegetables in the basket. Cover, turn heat to high, and steam the vegetables until they are tender but still hold their shape when pierced with a fork or knife. Check to make sure there is enough water in the saucepan as vegetables steam.

While the vegetables are steaming, whisk together the vinegar, olive oil, herbs, and shallot in a large bowl. Add the cooked vegetables to the dressing and gently toss. Add salt and pepper. Refrigerate 1 hour or overnight. Toss again before serving.

Cucumber-Seaweed Salad

Serves 4

Ranging in color from brown to dark green, the sea vegetable wakame is a potent source of iodine, which is critical to the production of thyroid hormone. Most of us are iodine deficient, which, as I wrote in The Thyroid Connection, *is a leading cause of the thyroid disease epidemic we are experiencing as a nation.*

Salad

- ¾ ounce dried wakame seaweed, cut into 1-inch pieces
- 2 cucumbers, peeled, seeded, and diced

Dressing

- 2 tablespoons apple cider vinegar
- 1½ tablespoons coconut aminos
- 1 tablespoon extra virgin olive oil
- Juice of ½ small lemon
- ½-inch piece of fresh ginger, peeled and grated
- Pinch of fine sea salt

In a bowl, soak the wakame in warm water for 5 to 10 minutes. Drain in a colander. Combine the seaweed and cucumber in a bowl.

In another bowl, whisk together the vinegar, coconut aminos, olive oil, lemon juice, ginger, and salt. Toss the vegetables with 2 tablespoons dressing. Taste and add more dressing if desired.

7

Main Courses

The perfect burgers. Pulled pork that almost falls apart by itself. Lean yet rich bison chili. Flank steak with an Asian twist. Comforting turkey pot pie. Herb roasted chicken. Halibut with lemon and capers. This chapter includes easy-to-prepare main courses for every palate and preference—along with tips to make preparation even easier (say hello to the Instant Pot!). Best of all, they are bursting with nutrients to jumpstart your health and reverse autoimmunity. So dig in!

When you're whipping up these amazing meals, remember to choose grass-fed, pasture-raised meats and poultry and wild-caught seafood for maximum health benefits without the GMOs, hormones, and antibiotics found in conventionally raised meat, poultry, and fish.

Herb Roasted Chicken

Serves 6

This is a variation of the roasted chicken my mom made when I was growing up. It warms my heart to carry on the tradition with my daughter. I roast a chicken at least once a week, and my family enjoys it for several days. If you don't have all the herbs on hand, feel free to substitute more or less of what you do have. There are always plenty of leftovers to add to salads, soups, and other dishes. Be sure to save the bones to make Gut-Healing Bone Broth (page 71).

1 4- to 5-pound whole organic, free-range chicken, giblets removed

1 tablespoon avocado oil

1 tablespoon fresh thyme

1 tablespoon fresh rosemary

1 teaspoon garlic powder

½ teaspoon freshly ground black pepper

¼ teaspoon fine sea salt

½ teaspoon celery seed

1 onion, chopped

2 garlic cloves

1 small lemon, sliced

½ cup Gut-Healing Bone Broth (page 71)

Pat the chicken dry and place in baking dish. Rub the chicken all over with the avocado oil.

In a bowl, combine thyme, rosemary, garlic powder, pepper, salt, and celery seed. Rub the spice blend all over the chicken. Stuff the onion, garlic, and lemon slices into the chicken cavity.

To make in an Instant Pot: Put the chicken and bone broth in the Instant Pot. Secure the lid, set to "Meat" and the timer to 30 minutes. Press "Start." When the timer goes off, let the Instant Pot naturally release pressure. This may take up to 15 to 20 minutes. Transfer the chicken from the Instant Pot to a platter. Let the chicken sit at room temperature for 10 minutes before carving.

To oven roast the chicken: Heat oven to 425°F. Roast in the oven for 1 hour or until a meat thermometer inserted in the thickest part reads 165°F. Let the chicken sit at room temperature for 10 minutes before carving.

Baked Chicken and Sweet Potatoes with Lemon-Rosemary Sauce

Serves 4

This all-in-one dish is simple to put together. Chicken breasts, chopped sweet potatoes, onion, and lemon slices are layered in a baking dish, and a lemon-rosemary vinaigrette is poured on it. While it's baking, prepare the Winter Salad with Maple Vinaigrette (page 145).

4 organic, free-range boneless, skinless chicken breasts

2 sweet potatoes, chopped into 1-inch cubes

½ red onion, thinly sliced

1 large lemon, thinly sliced

Juice of 1 large lemon

⅓ cup avocado oil

2 garlic cloves, minced

1 tablespoon fresh rosemary

⅛ teaspoon fine sea salt

⅛ teaspoon freshly ground black pepper

Heat oven to 400°F. Place chicken breasts in a baking dish large enough to hold them in a single layer. Top the chicken with the sweet potatoes, onion, and lemon slices.

In a bowl, whisk together lemon juice, avocado oil, garlic, rosemary, salt, and pepper. Pour the mixture over the chicken and vegetables.

Bake for 1 hour or until chicken and potatoes are cooked through (see page 56 for the proper internal temperature of chicken).

Chicken Rollatini with Bacon and Pesto

Serves 4

Thin chicken breasts are filled with pesto and wrapped with bacon. Once cooked, they are sliced into pinwheels. Serve with Broccolini with Garlic and Lemon (page 192) or use any leftover bacon fat in the pan to make Wilted Greens with Bacon (page 193).

4 organic, free-range boneless, skinless chicken breasts, pounded to ¼-inch thickness
8 slices pastured and nitrate-free bacon

½ cup Spinach-Kale Pesto (page 196)
1 tablespoon avocado oil

Heat oven to 400°F. Arrange chicken breasts on a work surface. Place 2 slices of bacon lengthwise on each chicken breast. Flip each chicken breast over and spread on 1 to 2 tablespoons pesto. Roll the chicken breasts up tightly with the bacon on the outside.

In a cast-iron skillet, heat the avocado oil over medium-high heat. Add the chicken breasts and sear until brown all over. Place the skillet in the oven for 10 minutes or until the internal temperature of the chicken reaches 165°F. Let the chicken breasts rest for 5 minutes before slicing.

Chicken Nuggets

Serves 4

Kids and adults alike will go crazy over these crispy chicken bites. I don't recommend consuming fried food regularly, however, as a special treat a few times a year is okay. Follow these few tips to guarantee that your chicken will be perfectly fried: Make sure the cooking oil is hot. Fry the chicken as soon as it's twice dredged in coconut milk and the flour mixture, or else the crunchy outer layer will become soggy. The chicken will also become soggy if the skillet is overcrowded and the oil temperature drops. Serve with Sweet Potato Fries (page 185) and Tangy Coleslaw (page 147). Serve with Ketchup (page 199) or Ranch Dressing (page 206) for dipping.

1 cup cassava flour

2 teaspoons onion powder

2 teaspoons garlic powder

1 teaspoon freshly ground
    black pepper

¼ teaspoon fine sea salt

1 cup full-fat coconut milk

¼ cup avocado oil or coconut oil,
    for frying

1 pound organic, free-range
    boneless, skinless chicken
    breasts, cut into 1-inch pieces

In a shallow bowl, whisk together the cassava flour, onion and garlic powders, pepper, and salt. Pour the coconut milk into a separate shallow bowl.

In a deep skillet, heat the oil over medium-high heat. To check that oil is hot, dip the end of a wooden spoon into oil and if it bubbles, it is ready.

Dip each piece of chicken into the coconut milk, then into the flour mixture. Repeat for a second coat.

When the oil is hot, gently add the chicken to the skillet. Cook 3 to 4 minutes on each side, until the nuggets are crispy. Drain the nuggets on a paper towel–lined plate and serve hot.

Chicken Pad Thai

Serves 4

Thai, Vietnamese, and Chinese are some of my favorite flavors. Luckily, we can all still enjoy this traditional Thai dish using coconut aminos, coconut milk, and sweet potato and carrot "noodles." Feel free to experiment and substitute the chicken with shrimp, beef, or pork.

1 tablespoon avocado oil

½ red onion, chopped

1 garlic clove, minced

1 sweet potato, spiralized or julienned

2 carrots, spiralized or julienned

1 pound organic, free-range boneless, skinless chicken breasts, sliced into 1-inch pieces

¼ cup "Peanut" Sauce (page 201)

½ cup coconut aminos

1 cup thinly sliced red cabbage

¼ cup chopped cilantro, for garnish

2 green onions, thinly sliced, for garnish

1 lime, quartered

In a skillet, sauté the onion and garlic in avocado oil over medium heat until translucent. Add the sweet potatoes and carrots and sauté until soft, approximately 5 minutes. Transfer the vegetables to a plate.

Add the chicken to the same skillet and cook, stirring frequently until cooked through, about 5 to 8 minutes.

While the chicken is cooking, whisk together the "Peanut" Sauce and coconut aminos in a bowl. Add the sauce and the cooked vegetables to the skillet. Add the cabbage and cook, stirring frequently, for 2 minutes until the cabbage is wilted but still firm. Divide among four plates. Garnish with cilantro, green onions, and lime wedges.

Chicken Burrito Bowl

Serves 4

Finding creative ways to make delicious and autoimmune-friendly Mexican food has become a passion of mine. When I first served this dish to my husband's parents, my mother-in-law asked for the recipe. What a compliment! The cilantro, lime juice, and cumin add lively Mexican flavors to Cauliflower Rice (page 67).

2 tablespoons avocado oil

2 garlic cloves, minced

4 cups Cauliflower Rice (page 67)

1 cup cilantro leaves

Juice of 1 lime

1 pound organic, free-range boneless, skinless chicken breasts, cut into 1-inch pieces

2 teaspoons ground cumin

¼ teaspoon fine sea salt

2 zucchinis, chopped into 1-inch pieces

2 cups sliced mushrooms

1 onion, thinly sliced

1 cup Five-Vegetable Guacamole (page 220)

In a skillet, add 1 tablespoon avocado oil and garlic. Sauté over medium-high heat until the garlic is just fragrant (it doesn't take long!), taking care so it doesn't burn. Add the Cauliflower Rice and sauté for 5 minutes, until soft. Stir in the cilantro and lime juice and transfer to a bowl.

Season the chicken with the cumin and salt. Add 1 tablespoon avocado oil to the same skillet. When hot, add the chicken. Sauté for 5 to 7 minutes, until cooked through. Transfer the chicken to a plate.

Add the zucchinis, mushrooms, and onions to the skillet and cook for 4 to 6 minutes, until softened. Season with salt and pepper. Divide the Cauliflower Rice and vegetables between four bowls. Top with the cooked chicken and accompany with the guacamole on the side.

Turkey Pot Pie

Serves 4

This is another hearty, comfort-food classic dish that all of us can now enjoy thanks to cassava and coconut flours. They're combined with a bit of gelatin to make a biscuit-like topping. Feel free to use ground chicken, lamb, or beef, or a meat mixture, in place of the turkey if you prefer.

Filling

- 2 slices pastured and nitrate-free bacon, chopped
- 1 pound organic ground turkey
- ½ onion, chopped
- 1 leek, chopped
- 3 garlic cloves, grated or minced
- 1 cup sliced baby bella or other mushrooms
- 3 cups cubed butternut squash
- 4 cups packed kale leaves, torn into small pieces
- ½ teaspoon fine sea salt
- ½ teaspoon freshly ground black pepper
- 3 cups Gut-Healing Bone Broth (page 71)

Biscuit Topping

- ¾ cup cassava flour
- ¼ cup coconut flour
- 1 tablespoon The Myers Way Gelatin (or similar gelatin)
- ¼ teaspoon baking soda
- ¼ teaspoon cream of tartar
- ¼ teaspoon fine sea salt
- 1 tablespoon coconut oil
- 1 cup filtered water

Heat oven to 375°F. Cook the bacon in a large skillet over medium-high heat. Once the bacon has rendered its fat, add the turkey and sauté, stirring frequently, until cooked through. Leaving the drippings in the skillet, use a slotted spoon to transfer the bacon and turkey to a bowl.

Add the onions, leeks, and garlic to the skillet and sauté for 5 minutes, until soft. Stir in the mushrooms, squash, kale, salt, and pepper and cook for

5 minutes, until vegetables soften. Add the bone broth, turkey, and bacon and stir well. Bring to a boil, then lower the heat to a simmer and cook for 10 minutes.

While the vegetables are cooking, make the biscuit topping. Whisk together the cassava and coconut flours, gelatin, baking soda, cream of tartar, and sea salt in the bowl of a mixer. Add the coconut oil, then turn the machine on low and slowly add the water. Mix until the dough holds together and is well combined. Pour the turkey-vegetable mixture into a 9-by-13-inch baking dish. Spoon heaping tablespoons of the biscuit topping onto the filling. Bake for 50 minutes. Let cool for 5 minutes before serving.

Mississippi Roast

Serves 6

In the early 2000s a woman in Mississippi put a chuck roast, a package of dry Ranch dressing, a package of dry gravy mix, and a stick of butter in her slow cooker. When the meat was done, it was flavorful and so tender it came apart like pulled pork. Since then, the recipe has become known as Mississippi Roast and has traveled across the internet to cooks everywhere. The Myers Way version uses dried herbs and spices instead of processed seasonings, and I add root vegetables for a complete meal.

2 pounds 100 percent grass-fed, pasture-raised chuck roast

½ cup Gut-Healing Bone Broth (page 71)

½ tablespoon dried parsley

½ tablespoon garlic powder

½ tablespoon onion powder

½ teaspoon fine sea salt

¼ teaspoon freshly ground black pepper

1 onion, chopped into 1-inch pieces

6 carrots, chopped into 1-inch pieces

2 rutabagas or turnips, chopped into 1-inch pieces

To make in an Instant Pot: Add the chuck roast, bone broth, seasonings, and onion to the Instant Pot. Set to "Pressure Cook" and set timer for 50 minutes. When timer goes off, quick-release the pressure. Open the Instant Pot and add the carrots and rutabagas. Close the lid and set to "Pressure Cook" for an additional 10 minutes. Quick-release the pressure. Transfer the meat and vegetables to a platter. Allow to sit for 5 minutes, then slice and serve with the vegetables.

To cook in a slow cooker: Place all ingredients in a slow cooker and cook for 6 to 8 hours at high heat.

World's Best Asian Flank Steak

Serves 4

This is my favorite recipe in this cookbook for two reasons: it's absolutely the best flank steak in the world, and Xavier and I requested that this marinade be used on the beef tenderloins we served at our wedding. Flank steak takes to any kind of marinade, especially one with Southeast Asian ingredients. Once marinated, it's only minutes from pan to plate. I find endless ways to use this recipe: for dinner with some Grilled Bok Choy (page 194), as a salad for lunch with some Cucumber-Seaweed Salad (page 149), or on a bed of organic field greens.

½ cup coconut aminos

½ cup toasted sesame oil

2 tablespoons honey

2 garlic cloves, minced

2 tablespoons fish sauce

1 tablespoon grated fresh ginger

1 pound 100 percent grass-fed, pasture-raised flank steak

1 tablespoon avocado oil

1 bunch green onions, diagonally sliced, for garnish

In a baking dish, whisk together the coconut aminos, sesame oil, honey, garlic, fish sauce, and ginger. Add the flank steak to the marinade and marinate in the refrigerator for 1 hour, turning the meat every so often, or marinate overnight.

In a large skillet or grill pan, heat the avocado oil over medium-high heat. Add the flank steak and sear 4 minutes on each side (or to desired doneness). Transfer the steak to a cutting board and let it rest 5 minutes before slicing. Garnish with green onions.

The Perfect Fast Man Burgers

Serves 4

My dad (aka The Fast Man) was an incredible cook. He was particularly known for his perfectly grilled hamburgers. This is my adaptation of his burgers. Although I give instructions for cooking the burgers in a grill pan, feel free to use an outdoor grill (which is how my dad always grilled them). You can double or triple this recipe and enjoy these burgers at a backyard barbecue with Tangy Coleslaw (page 147), Root Vegetable Chips (page 215), and any of the toppings listed below.

1 pound 100 percent grass-fed, pasture-raised ground beef

1 tablespoon Gut-Healing Bone Broth (page 71)

1 tablespoon garlic powder

1 tablespoon onion powder

1 teaspoon dried thyme

1 teaspoon freshly ground black pepper

½ teaspoon fine sea salt

Optional Toppings

Five-Vegetable Guacamole (page 220)

Rutabaga "Hummus" (page 217)

Grilled pineapple

Caramelized Onions (page 72)

Ketchup (page 199)

Mustard (made with apple cider vinegar)

Place all burger ingredients in a bowl. Using clean hands, mix together well. Shape into four patties.

Heat a grill pan or skillet over high heat. Grill the burgers on one side for 4 to 6 minutes. Turn the burgers and grill on the other side for about 5 minutes, or to desired doneness. Serve with toppings of your choice.

Meatballs

Serves 4

The basil, thyme, and sea salt in this recipe make these meatballs mouthwatering. Pair with Zucchini Noodles with Spinach-Kale Pesto (page 196) for a spin on meatballs and spaghetti.

1 small yellow onion, coarsely chopped

½ cup fresh basil leaves

1 cup grated zucchini

2 teaspoons dried thyme

2 teaspoons fine sea salt

1 pound 100 percent grass-fed, pasture-raised ground beef

Heat oven to 375°F. Line a sheet pan with parchment paper.

Place onion, basil, zucchini, thyme, and salt in a food processor or blender. Pulse until coarsely chopped.

Combine the mixture with the ground beef. Using clean hands, mix well until blended. Shape into meatballs of equal size, using approximately 1 to 2 tablespoons of meat for each. Arrange the meatballs on the sheet pan about 1 inch apart.

Bake for 25 minutes, or until cooked through in the center. Once cooked, remove from oven and serve.

Bison Chili

Serves 4

Bison (buffalo) is flavorful and protein-rich and lower in total fat and cholesterol than beef, chicken, turkey, and pork. Many supermarkets carry grass-fed, pasture-raised ground bison. Or, you can find bison ranchers online who can deliver a variety of bison cuts like roasts and ribs to your door. If you can't find bison locally, substitute ground beef in this recipe.

8 carrots, peeled and chopped

8 celery stalks, chopped

1 onion, chopped

2 garlic cloves, grated or minced

1 beet, peeled and chopped

1 pound 100 percent grass-fed, pasture-raised ground bison

1 tablespoon fresh oregano

1 teaspoon ground cumin

1 teaspoon fine sea salt

3 cups Gut-Healing Bone Broth (page 71)

1 bunch cilantro, chopped, for garnish

1 avocado, sliced

To make in an Instant Pot: Set the Instant Pot to "Sauté." When hot, add carrots, celery, onion, garlic, and beet and sauté for 5 minutes. Stir in the bison, oregano, cumin, and salt, breaking up the meat with a wooden spoon. When the bison is no longer raw, add the broth, and close the Instant Pot. Press "Cancel," change the setting to "Stew/Chili," and set the timer for 30 minutes. When the timer goes off, quick-release the pressure. Divide the chili among four bowls and top with cilantro and avocado.

To make on the stove: In a Dutch oven or large pot, add the carrots, celery, onion, garlic, and beet and sauté for 5 minutes. Stir in the bison, oregano, cumin, and salt, breaking up the meat with a wooden spoon. When the bison is no longer raw, add the broth. Bring to a boil, then reduce to a simmer for 30 minutes while flavors develop. Divide chili among four bowls and top with cilantro and avocado.

Lamb Chops with Cherry Glaze

Serves 2

These lamb chops are broiled (they can also be grilled outdoors) and then brushed with a sweet-and-sour cherry glaze. Pair them with Brussels Sprouts and Red Cabbage Salad (page 142) or Broccolini with Garlic and Lemon (page 192). I keep an extra bowl of the glaze on the table for dipping. Store any glaze leftovers in the refrigerator to brush over pork chops or chicken before grilling.

Glaze
- 1 cup cherries
- ¾ cup Gut-Healing Bone Broth (page 71)
- 2 teaspoons apple cider vinegar
- 2 teaspoons honey
- 1 tablespoon tapioca starch

Lamb
- 4 ½-inch-thick 100 percent grass-fed, pasture-raised lamb chops
- 2 tablespoons avocado oil
- 2 tablespoons fresh rosemary leaves
- 1 teaspoon minced garlic
- ½ teaspoon fine sea salt
- ½ teaspoon freshly ground black pepper

To make the glaze: In a saucepan at medium-high heat, combine the cherries, ½ cup bone broth, apple cider vinegar, and honey. Bring to a boil, and then lower the heat to a simmer for 8 minutes, stirring occasionally. In a separate bowl, add ¼ cup bone broth and tapioca starch. Whisk together. Once combined, pour into saucepan and stir until sauce thickens.

To make the lamb chops: Turn the oven to broil. Brush the avocado oil on the chops. Combine seasonings and press evenly onto chops. Place chops in a baking dish and broil for 5 to 6 minutes on each side. Transfer lamb to a plate and let rest for 5 minutes. Top with cherry glaze and serve.

Pesto Pizza

Serves 2

Who doesn't love pizza? This will be a favorite for sure! The pizza crust comes out of the oven thin and crisp. Use just about any thinly sliced vegetable as a topping with pesto or tomato-free No-Mato Sauce (page 198).

Dough

2/3 cup arrowroot flour

1/4 cup cassava flour

2 tablespoons tigernut flour

1 teaspoon cream of tartar

1/2 teaspoon baking soda

1/2 teaspoon fine sea salt

2 tablespoons extra virgin olive oil

1/2 cup warm filtered water

Topping

1/2 cup Spinach-Kale Pesto
(page 196)

Suggested toppings: Arugula,
sliced olives, sliced zucchini,
sliced squash, spinach,
fresh basil

Heat oven to 425°F. In a mixing bowl, whisk together the arrowroot flour, cassava flour, tigernut flour, cream of tartar, baking soda, and salt. Stir in the olive oil. Slowly add warm water to the bowl, and using clean hands, mix until a ball forms.

Place the dough on a sheet pan or pizza stone. Roll out the dough to a 1/4-inch thickness. Bake for 8 minutes or until brown.

Remove crust from the oven and top with the pesto and other desired toppings. Turn the oven to broil and return the pizza to the oven. Broil for 2 to 3 minutes, keeping an eye on the toppings to make sure they don't burn. Remove the pizza from the oven and let it sit for a few minutes before slicing.

Pesto Pizza, page 166

Braised Pork Ribs with
Cherry Barbecue Sauce, pages 171 and 200

Grilled Bok Choy, page 194

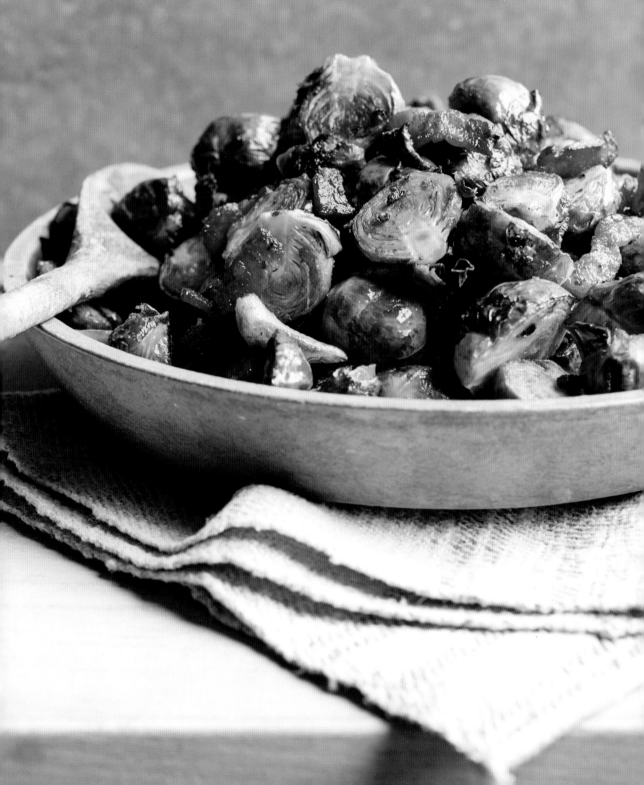

Roasted Brussels Sprouts with Bacon, page 187

Chicken Pad Thai, page 156

Aïoli, page 197

No-Mato Sauce, page 198

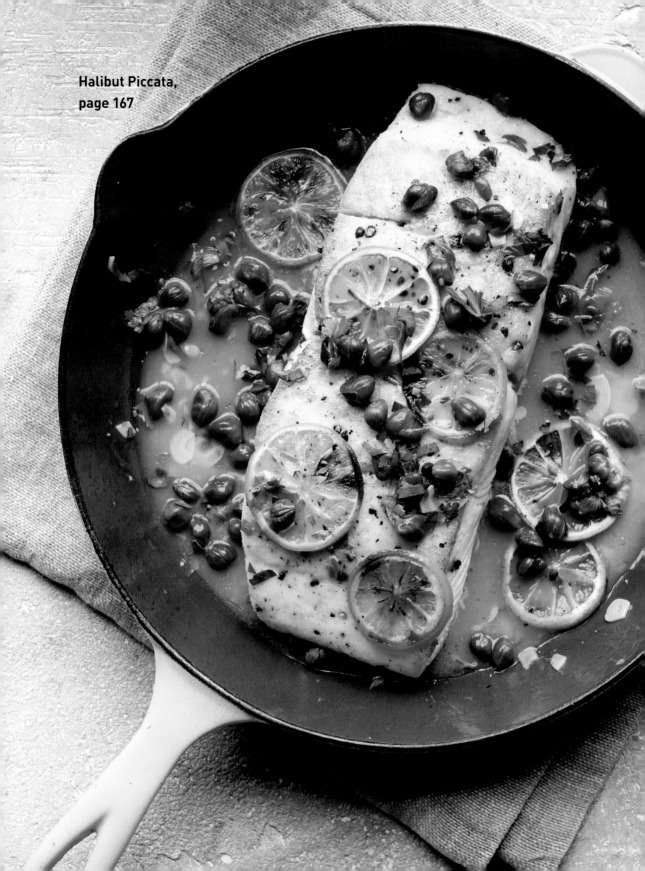

Halibut Piccata,
page 167

Halibut Piccata

Serves 4

This recipe uses halibut, and cod or other fish fillets would also work. The quick pan sauce is made with some broth, capers, and lemon juice. Broccolini with Garlic and Lemon (page 192) or a salad of dark, leafy greens with Betty's Italian Dressing (page 205) completes this Italian meal.

1 tablespoon avocado oil

¼ cup cassava flour

4 4- to 6-ounce wild-caught
   halibut fillets

2 cloves garlic, minced

1½ cups Gut-Healing Bone Broth
   (page 71), divided

½ cup freshly squeezed
   lemon juice

1 tablespoon arrowroot flour

1 heaping tablespoon capers,
   rinsed and drained

Chopped parsley for garnish

In a skillet, heat the avocado oil over medium-high heat.

Put the cassava flour in a shallow bowl and lightly coat the halibut fillets on both sides. Add the halibut to the skillet and cook for 6 minutes. Turn the fish and cook for another 6 minutes. Transfer the fish to a plate.

To the same skillet, add the garlic and sauté until fragrant. Whisk in 1 cup bone broth and the lemon juice. In a bowl, whisk together the arrowroot flour and the remaining ½ cup broth. Add to the skillet and whisk to combine. Add the capers and return the halibut to the skillet to heat through. Garnish with chopped parsley.

Pork Tenderloin with Mustard Sauce

Serves 4

One pan, four ingredients. This easy pork dish comes together in minutes. Pair with Loaded and Baked Sweet Potatoes (page 191) and a salad of arugula, Belgian endive, and a simple vinaigrette. Use a mustard made with apple cider vinegar rather than distilled vinegar.

1 pound pasture-raised pork
   tenderloin
½ cup Gut-Healing Bone Broth
   (page 71)

2 tablespoons Dijon mustard
1 teaspoon arrowroot flour

Heat oven to 350°F. In an ovenproof skillet over high heat, sear the pork tenderloin for 3 to 4 minutes on all sides.

Place the skillet in the oven and roast the pork for 10 minutes, or until it reaches an internal temperature of 150°F. Remove the pan from the oven and transfer the pork to a cutting board. Let sit for 5 to 10 minutes, then slice into ½-inch pieces.

In the same skillet over medium heat, whisk together the broth and mustard. Bring to a boil, then lower the heat to a simmer. Stir in the arrowroot flour, constantly whisking and cooking until the sauce is thickened and there are no lumps. Serve the sauce over the sliced pork.

Carolina Pulled Pork

Serves 4

Meltingly tender, once cooked the meat just falls apart at the slightest poke of a fork. Pair with Tangy Coleslaw (page 147) or Wilted Greens with Bacon (page 193) to complete this Southern classic.

2 pounds pasture-raised
pork butt
Meat Marinade (page 202)

½ cup Gut-Healing Bone Broth
(page 71)
¼ cup apple cider vinegar

In a baking dish or bowl, marinate pork butt in marinade for 1 hour or overnight.

To make in an Instant Pot: Discard the marinade. Put the pork in Instant Pot with bone broth and apple cider vinegar. Set to "Meat" and cook for 60 minutes. Quick-release the pressure, and shred the pork with two forks.

To make in a slow cooker: Place all ingredients in slow cooker and cook for 5 hours on low. Discard the marinade, transfer to a serving platter, and shred the pork with two forks.

To make in the oven: Heat oven to 300°F. In a Dutch oven, sear the pork butt over medium-high heat, about 3 to 5 minutes on all sides. Add the broth and apple cider vinegar. Cover and bake for 3 hours. Discard the marinade, transfer to a serving platter, and shred the pork with two forks.

Apple-Stuffed Pork Chops with Maple Glaze

Serves 4

A fun way to dress up pork chops is with this easy apple stuffing. Pair with Roasted Brussels Sprouts with Bacon (page 187) or Mashed Cauliflower and Rutabaga (page 189). Round out the meal with a salad of organic dark leafy greens, such as kale, escarole, and spinach.

4 bone-in pasture-raised organic pork chops	1 tablespoon avocado oil
¾ cup Gut-Healing Bone Broth (page 71), divided	1 Granny Smith apple, peeled and diced
½ cup maple syrup	½ onion, chopped
1 tablespoon tapioca starch	1 garlic clove, minced

Heat oven to 350°F. Cut a pocket for stuffing in each chop by slicing from the fat side almost to the bone.

To make the glaze: In a saucepan, heat ¼ cup bone broth and maple syrup over medium heat. In a separate bowl, whisk together ¼ cup bone broth and tapioca starch. Add the starch mixture to the saucepan and stir until sauce thickens. Set aside.

To make the filling: To a skillet over medium-high heat, add avocado oil and sauté apple, onion, and garlic until the apple is soft. Transfer to a bowl and cool until cool enough to handle.

Stuff each pork chop with filling. Carefully add pork chops to the same skillet, sear on both sides, about 3 to 4 minutes, and then brush with some of the glaze. Add the remaining filling and the remaining ¼ cup bone broth to the skillet.

Place skillet in the oven and bake for 15 to 20 minutes, brushing with glaze every 5 minutes, until the pork reaches an internal temperature of 150°F. Divide the chops among four plates and spoon on the remaining glaze and filling.

Braised Pork Ribs

Serves 2

When I was growing up I never much cared for barbecue, however, once I moved to Texas and started eating red meat, I became addicted to it. Unfortunately, lots of commercial barbecue sauces contain sugar and preservatives so I learned to make my own. To make this dish, you can use any style of pork ribs—baby backs, spare ribs, riblets, country style. Serve with Tangy Coleslaw (page 147) and Sweet Potato Biscuits (page 102).

2–3 pounds pasture-raised
  pork ribs

1 cup Cherry Barbecue Sauce
  (page 200)

1 cup Gut-Healing Bone Broth
  (page 71)

2 tablespoons coconut aminos

1 tablespoon honey

At the end of the rack of ribs, slide a dinner knife under the membrane and lift it up. Grab the membrane with a paper towel, pull it off, and discard.

In a bowl, whisk together barbeque sauce, bone broth, coconut aminos, and honey.

To make in an Instant Pot: Place the ribs in an Instant Pot and add the sauce. Set to "Meat" and set the timer for 20 minutes. When the meat is finished, slow release pressure for 5 minutes, then quick-release remaining pressure. Heat the oven to broil. Transfer the ribs, but not the sauce, to a parchment paper–lined sheet pan. Set the Instant Pot to "Sauté" and cook the sauce for about 5 minutes, until thickened. Brush the sauce on the ribs and broil for 5 minutes.

To make in a slow cooker: Place all ingredients in a slow cooker and cook on low for 8 hours.

To make in the oven: Heat oven to 300°F. Line a sheet pan with parchment paper. Set a rack on top of the pan. Set oven to broil on high. Brush the pork lightly with sauce. Put the pork, meaty side up, on the rack and broil 5 minutes. Return oven to 300°F. Brush half the sauce onto ribs and bake for 1½ to 2 hours, brushing with remaining sauce every 20 to 30 minutes.

Honey-Ginger Glazed Salmon

Serves 2

Xavier and I make this simple salmon dish once a week. Salmon is filled with healthy anti-inflammatory omega-3 fatty acids, and the ginger helps to reduce inflammation. Serve with Broccolini with Garlic and Lemon (page 192) or Roasted Vegetables (page 183).

¼ cup coconut aminos

¼ cup toasted sesame oil

1 tablespoon honey

2 garlic cloves, grated or minced

1 teaspoon ginger, grated or minced

2 4- to 6-ounce wild-caught salmon fillets

1 green onion, thinly sliced, for garnish

Heat oven to 375°F. In a baking dish, whisk together the coconut aminos, sesame oil, honey, garlic, and ginger. Add the salmon and marinate in the refrigerator for 30 minutes.

Place the salmon in the oven and bake for 25 minutes.

Turn the oven to broil. Place the baking dish under the broiler for 2 to 3 minutes, until salmon is browned. Garnish with the green onion before serving.

Lamb Meatballs in Lettuce Wraps

Serves 4

For these Mediterranean wraps, large lettuce leaves, in place of pita, are filled with tender and juicy lamb meatballs, cucumbers, and olives with a drizzle of Tzatziki (page 204).

1 pound 100 percent grass-fed, pasture-raised ground lamb

1 shallot, minced

2 garlic cloves, minced

2 tablespoons lemon juice

1 teaspoon dried oregano

½ teaspoon ground cumin

¼ teaspoon freshly ground black pepper

⅛ teaspoon fine sea salt

1 tablespoon avocado oil

1 onion, thinly sliced

8 lettuce leaves—Bibb, romaine, or other large leaves

1 cucumber, quartered and thinly sliced

About 15 Kalamata olives, pitted and sliced

Tzatziki (page 204)

Heat oven to 350°F. Line a sheet pan with parchment paper.

In a bowl, combine lamb, shallot, garlic, lemon juice, oregano, cumin, pepper, and salt. Using clean hands, mix well and shape into 1-inch balls. Arrange the meatballs on the prepared sheet pan and bake for 25 minutes.

While the meatballs cook, heat the avocado oil in a skillet over medium heat. Add the onion and cook slowly, stirring occasionally, until they are caramelized, 25 to 30 minutes (see page 72).

Transfer meatballs from the oven and let sit for 5 minutes. Arrange the meatballs, caramelized onions, lettuce leaves, cucumber, and olives on a platter. To eat, place some meatballs, onions, cucumber, and olives on a lettuce leaf, then top with tzatziki, wrap up, and enjoy!

Create Your Own Coconut Curry

Serves 6

Curries—warming and inviting—remind me of my time in India. You can change up the ingredients of this versatile dish to your liking. It's best to make your own spice blends, since many commercial ones contain nightshade vegetables. Doing so also allows you to add more cinnamon or less cumin, for instance, to suit your taste. Keep the dish vegetarian or add beef, pork, chicken, or shrimp. Or replace the vegetables listed below with others, such as cauliflower, butternut squash, and carrots. Spoon it over Cauliflower Rice (page 67) or Cauliflower Saffron "Rice" (page 188). Enjoy the leftovers for lunch the next day.

1 tablespoon avocado oil

1 onion, chopped

3 cloves garlic, minced

1 head broccoli, cut into florets

1 sweet potato, peeled and
   cubed

2 cups Gut-Healing Bone Broth
   (page 71)

2 cups full-fat coconut milk

1 tablespoon grated fresh ginger

1 teaspoon ground cinnamon

1 tablespoon ground turmeric

1 teaspoon ground cumin

1 teaspoon freshly ground
   black pepper

½ teaspoon fine sea salt

2 tablespoons arrowroot flour
   (optional)

1 cup chopped cilantro,
   for garnish

To make in an Instant Pot: Set the Instant Pot to "Sauté." Once heated, add the avocado oil, onions, and garlic. Sauté until the onions are translucent. Add the broccoli and sweet potato and sauté for 5 minutes. Add the remaining ingredients, except the cilantro, and press "Cancel." Cover the Instant Pot and set on "Soup" setting. Reset timer to 10 minutes and press "Start." Once finished, quick-release the pressure. Remove the lid and add the arrowroot flour; stir to thicken. Serve in bowls and garnish with cilantro.

To make on the stovetop: In a Dutch oven, heat the oil, onions, and garlic over medium heat. Sauté until the onions are translucent. Add the broccoli and sweet potato and cook for 5 minutes, stirring frequently. Add the bone broth, coconut milk, ginger, cinnamon, turmeric, cumin, pepper, and salt. Simmer for 10 minutes. Stir in the arrowroot flour to thicken the sauce. Serve in bowls and garnish with cilantro.

Coconut Shrimp

Serves 4

When I was growing up in New Orleans, my grandparents took the family out to dinner at the Yacht Club for special occasions, and I always ordered a fried shrimp po'boy—a traditional Louisiana sandwich. This substitute for fried shrimp is a healthier option that everyone will love. The shrimp are tossed with coconut flour and shredded coconut instead of breadcrumbs—and they are so easy to make! Double or triple the recipe for a party appetizer. My husband and I served this as an appetizer at our wedding.

2 tablespoons coconut flour

½ cup unsweetened shredded coconut

1 teaspoon garlic powder

1 teaspoon onion powder

½ teaspoon fine sea salt

½ teaspoon freshly ground black pepper

¾ cup full-fat coconut milk

1½ tablespoons coconut aminos

1 pound wild-caught shrimp

Heat oven to 400°F. In a shallow bowl, whisk together coconut flour, shredded coconut, garlic and onion powders, salt, and pepper.

In another shallow bowl, whisk together the coconut milk and coconut aminos.

Dip each shrimp into the liquid mixture, and then into the dry mixture to coat. Arrange in a single layer in a baking dish. Bake for 15 to 20 minutes, until golden brown. For extra crispiness, remove the pan and set the oven to broil. Broil the shrimp for 4 to 5 minutes.

Vegetable Fried "Rice"

Serves 2

Cauliflower Rice (page 67) again shows its versatility in this colorful vegetable medley. You can substitute other vegetables of your choosing or top it with some leftover grilled chicken, pork, or shrimp to make a complete meal. This fried "rice" also makes the perfect accompaniment with thin slices of the World's Best Asian Flank Steak (page 161).

1 tablespoon avocado oil

½ onion, chopped

3 garlic cloves, grated or minced

1 zucchini, shredded

2 carrots, finely chopped

2 cups Cauliflower Rice (page 67)

2 tablespoons coconut aminos

1 tablespoon fish sauce

3 tablespoons toasted sesame oil

1 cup shredded red cabbage

½ teaspoon fine sea salt

Freshly ground black pepper, to taste

2 green onions, thinly sliced, for garnish

Heat the avocado oil in a skillet over medium-high heat; then add onion and garlic and sauté until the onion is translucent. Add zucchini, carrots, and Cauliflower Rice. Sauté for 5 minutes.

In a separate bowl, whisk together coconut aminos, fish sauce, and sesame oil. Add to vegetable mixture and combine. Once the carrots are cooked through, add the cabbage and cook, stirring frequently, until wilted but still crisp. Add the salt and pepper. Divide between two plates and garnish with sliced green onions.

Chimichurri Lamb Kebobs

Serves 4

I first learned of chimichurri, the Argentinian equivalent of ketchup, while living in South America and traveling in Argentina. Chimichurri is bright green with herbs and is always served with grilled meats. When making kebobs, cut the meat and vegetables to the same size for even cooking.

8 wooden skewers

¼ cup extra virgin olive oil

½ cup apple cider vinegar

¼ cup fresh cilantro

¼ cup fresh parsley

2 cloves garlic

2 zucchinis, sliced

2 onions, cut into 1-inch pieces

1 pound 100 percent grass-fed, pasture-raised lamb loin, cut into 1½-inch cubes

1 tablespoon avocado oil

Soak the wooden skewers in water for 30 minutes (so they don't burn when you use them).

To make the chimichurri sauce: In a food processor or high-speed blender, combine the olive oil, apple cider vinegar, cilantro, parsley, and garlic. Pulse until the herbs are coarsely chopped.

To make the kebobs: Thread the zucchini, onion, and lamb onto the skewers. Heat a grill pan to medium heat, then brush the pan with the oil. Place kebobs on the pan and cook for 5 minutes on each side or until an instant-read meat thermometer inserted into the lamb reads 130°F for medium rare. Divide the skewers among four plates and spoon on the chimichurri sauce.

Mushroom and Asparagus Caulisotto

Serves 2

Caulisotto? What's that? It's my name for a risotto-like dish made with Cauli-flower Rice (page 67), mushrooms, and asparagus. Unlike traditional risotto, you don't have to stand and stir it for 30 minutes, and it has the added bonus of being grain-free! Carrots, spinach, celery, and even bits of nitrate-free bacon are good additions or substitutions. Serve as a main course or as a side dish with Herb Roasted Chicken (page 152) or any pork dish.

1 tablespoon avocado oil

½ onion, chopped

2 garlic cloves, grated

2 cups Cauliflower Rice (page 67)

10 to 15 spears asparagus, trimmed and chopped into 1-inch pieces

1 cup sliced mushrooms

½ cup Gut-Healing Bone Broth (page 71)

¼ cup full-fat coconut milk

¼ teaspoon freshly ground black pepper

¼ teaspoon coarse sea salt

Put the oil, onion, and garlic in a large saucepan or Dutch oven. Sauté over low heat about 5 or 6 minutes, until the onions are translucent. Add the Cauliflower Rice, asparagus, mushrooms, and bone broth. Cook for 3 minutes, then cover and simmer for another 5 minutes.

Add the coconut milk, pepper, and salt. Cook until the Cauliflower Rice has absorbed most of the liquid. The caulisotto should be creamy, not dry.

8

Sides

Side dishes deserve time in the spotlight too! In fact, these super-healing vegetable dishes can do double duty as either side dishes or main courses (just bulk up the portions!). Either way, you'll love the rich tastes and creative takes on these classic and modern dishes. Whether you choose Zucchini Noodles with Spinach-Kale Pesto (page 184), Roasted Brussels Sprouts with Bacon (page 187), Loaded and Baked Sweet Potatoes (page 191), or any of the other mouthwatering dishes, you can't go wrong with these delicious sides!

Bacon-Wrapped Asparagus

Serves 8

This is a simple, yet elegant, first course or accompaniment to grilled fish or chicken. It's a great recipe to have your children be involved in making. They can wrap the bacon around the asparagus and get dinner table praise for helping in the kitchen.

4 slices pastured and
    nitrate-free bacon
48 asparagus spears,
    trimmed

Fine sea salt and freshly ground
    pepper, to taste

Heat oven to 425°F. Cut slices of bacon in half. Separate asparagus into eight bundles of about 6 spears and wrap one piece of bacon around each.

Arrange in a single layer on a parchment paper–lined baking sheet. Season with salt and pepper.

Roast in oven for 25 minutes.

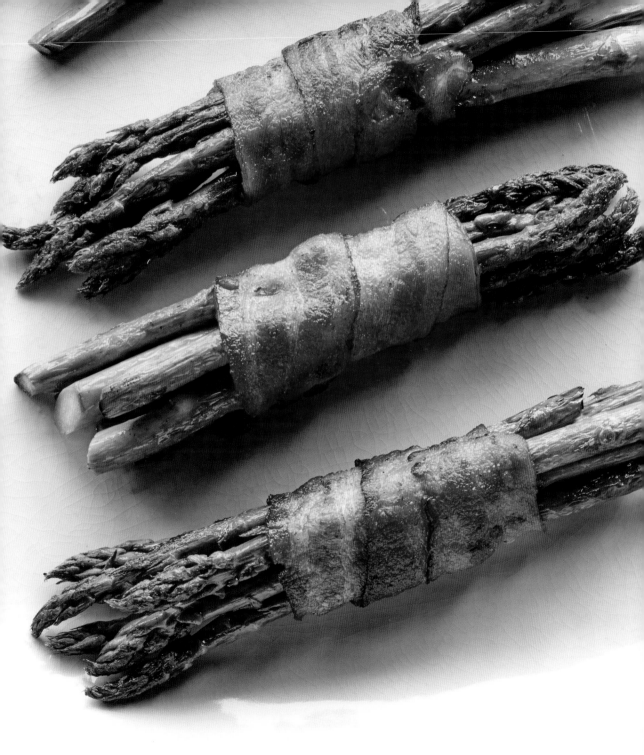

Bacon-Wrapped Asparagus, page 182

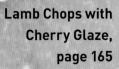

Lamb Chops with
Cherry Glaze,
page 165

Mushroom and
Asparagus
Caulisotto,
page 179

Wilted Greens with Bacon, page 193

Coconut Shrimp, page 176

Meatballs paired with Zucchini Noodles, pages 163 and 184

Mango-Avocado Salsa, page 210

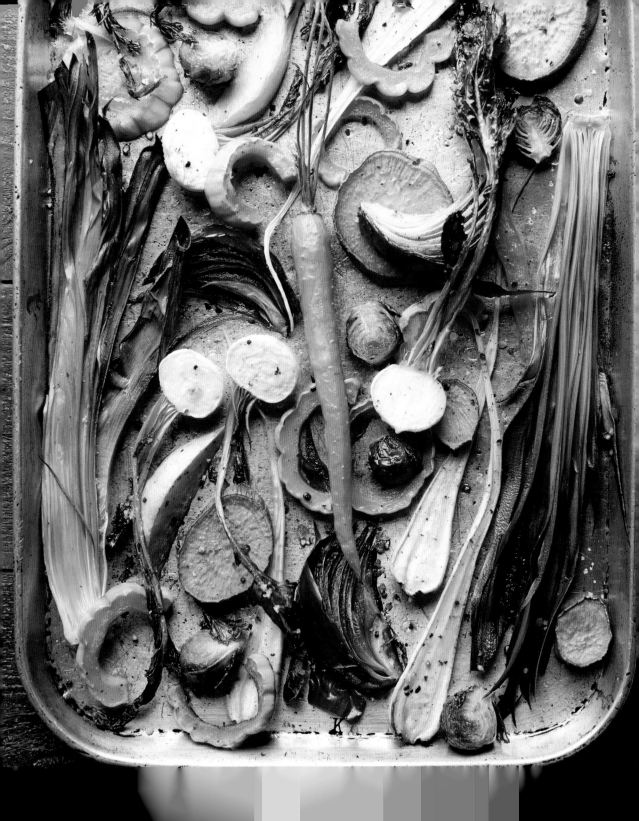

Roasted Vegetables

Serves 4

When making these crisp-on-the-outside, tender-on-the-inside vegetables, I often double the recipe. They go with just about any main course, but you can also pack them for lunch at work or when traveling. Some vegetables may require more time in the oven than others, depending on how they are sliced or chopped. Asparagus, green onions, and shallots can be left whole. Cut brussels sprouts, baby artichokes, and cauliflower and broccoli florets in half. Slice onions, summer squash, rutabaga, and sweet potatoes into ½-inch pieces. Slice parsnips and carrots into horizontal quarters, if large. Smaller ones can be left whole. Once roasted, sprinkle veggies with chopped herbs of your choosing. A platter of these beauties will disappear at any gathering.

1 pound vegetables, prepared as described above

2 tablespoons avocado oil

½ teaspoon fine sea salt

1 teaspoon freshly ground black pepper

Heat oven to 425°F. Line a sheet pan with parchment paper. Place vegetables on the pan and drizzle with avocado oil.

Using clean hands, toss to coat veggies with the oil. Arrange in a single layer and season with salt and pepper.

Bake for 10 to 15 minutes, turn the vegetables, and bake for another 10 to 15 minutes, or until crisp.

Zucchini Noodles with Spinach-Kale Pesto

Serves 2 as a side dish or 1 as a main dish

Make vegetable noodles with a spiralizer or a smaller, handy gadget called a julienne peeler. Just pull the peeler down the length of the zucchini or other vegetable, and you've got noodles! This recipe is quick to make and is perfect for a weeknight meal.

1 zucchini

1 tablespoon avocado oil

3 tablespoons Spinach-Kale Pesto (page 196)

Make zucchini noodles with a spiralizer following the manufacturer's instructions, or use a julienne peeler.

Heat the oil in a skillet over medium-high heat. Add the zucchini noodles and cook, tossing with tongs, for 1 to 2 minutes. Stir in the pesto and toss well to coat. Serve immediately.

Sweet Potato Fries

Serves 2

Kids and adults alike will love these sweet potato fries. These fries can be prepared with all kinds of root vegetables—carrots, parsnips, and yucca—or a combination. Change up the seasonings—a sprinkle of cinnamon or cumin instead of the garlic powder, for instance. Double or triple the amount you make for more people to enjoy. Serve these with The Perfect Fast Man Burgers (page 162) or Chicken Nuggets (page 155).

1 sweet potato, peeled and sliced lengthwise	½ teaspoon garlic powder
1 tablespoon avocado oil	Fine sea salt and freshly ground black pepper, to taste

Heat oven to 425°F. Line a sheet pan with parchment paper.

In a bowl, toss the sweet potato slices, avocado oil, garlic powder, salt, and pepper to coat. Arrange sweet potatoes on the prepared sheet pan.

Bake for 15 minutes, turn, and bake for another 15 minutes, until crisp and brown on both sides.

Root Vegetable Pancakes

Makes 4 pancakes

For these "potato" pancakes, a combination of sweet potatoes, parsnips, and beets takes the place of traditional white potatoes. The gelatin serves as a binder, since no eggs are used. Top the pancakes with smoked salmon or applesauce. Shred the vegetables using a box grater.

2 cups shredded sweet potato

1 cup shredded parsnips

1 cup shredded beets

½ cup onion, finely chopped

½ teaspoon fine sea salt

½ teaspoon freshly ground
black pepper

2 tablespoons cassava flour

1 tablespoon The Myers Way Gelatin
(or similar gelatin)

1 tablespoon cool filtered water

2 tablespoons boiling water

1 tablespoon avocado oil

In a bowl, toss together the sweet potato, parsnips, beets, onion, salt, pepper, and cassava flour.

In a separate bowl, combine gelatin with the cool water. Stir in the boiling water and whisk until frothy. Add the gelatin to sweet potato mixture and stir well.

Heat a skillet over medium heat. Add the avocado oil and coat the pan. Drop ¼ cup of the mixture into the skillet and flatten. Cook for about 2 minutes on each side. Continue for three more pancakes.

Roasted Brussels Sprouts with Bacon

Serves 4

When brussels sprouts are in season, we make this recipe or a variation a few times a week in our house. Vegetables roasted at a high temperature become crisp and caramelized. Brussels sprouts tossed with bits of bacon and a maple-mustard glaze go well with pork, poultry, and beef. Add this great dish to your Thanksgiving menu.

2 tablespoons avocado oil

2 tablespoons Dijon mustard

2 teaspoons maple syrup

2 garlic cloves, grated

1 teaspoon freshly ground
   black pepper

1 pound brussels sprouts,
   trimmed and halved

4 slices pastured and nitrate-free
   bacon, chopped

Heat oven to 400°F. Line a sheet pan with parchment paper.

In a bowl, whisk together the avocado oil, mustard, maple syrup, garlic, and black pepper. Add the brussels sprouts and bacon and toss well. Arrange the brussels sprouts in a single layer on the prepared pan.

Bake for 15 minutes, toss the sprouts, and bake for another 15 minutes, until crisp on the outsides and tender when pierced with a knife.

Cauliflower Saffron "Rice"

Serves 2

While in India, I was wowed by all the bright colors I saw everywhere. And colors have meaning there. Red shows wealth and power. Green symbolizes health and harvest. Saffron, a bright orange-yellow, signifies courage and self-lessness. Some Buddhist monks and nuns wear saffron robes. Saffron is also the color and the name of the world's most expensive spice. It's expensive because the tiny stigmas, or threads, of the saffron crocus have to be picked by hand. Use saffron sparingly; you don't need much to make this bright rice.

2 tablespoons Gut-Healing Bone Broth (page 71)

½ tablespoon saffron

1 tablespoon avocado oil

1 clove garlic, minced

½ onion, chopped

1 cup Cauliflower Rice (page 67)

In a bowl, combine bone broth and saffron. Let sit 5 to 20 minutes so the saffron will release its flavor (called *blooming*).

Heat avocado oil in a skillet over medium-high heat. Add the garlic and onion to the pan and sauté until the onion is translucent. Add the Cauliflower Rice and continue to sauté until cooked through, about 5 to 8 minutes. Add saffron and broth mixture to the pan and stir to evenly coat the Cauliflower Rice.

Mashed Cauliflower and Rutabaga

Serves 4

White potatoes aren't the only root vegetable you can mash for a great side dish. Substitute parsnips or carrots for the rutabaga or use a combination of vegetables in this healthy mash.

½ head cauliflower, cut into florets

2 cups peeled and chopped rutabaga

1 15-ounce can coconut cream

2 garlic cloves, roasted (page 73)

¼ teaspoon fine sea salt

½ teaspoon freshly ground black pepper

¼ cup chopped chives, for garnish

Add 1 inch of water to a large saucepan. Insert a steamer basket. Bring to a boil and place cauliflower and rutabaga onto steamer basket. Steam for 10 to 15 minutes, until the vegetables are tender when pierced with a knife. Remove steamer basket and pour water out of saucepan. Place vegetables back in saucepan.

Add the coconut cream, garlic, salt, and pepper. Bring to a boil then remove from heat.

For a coarse puree, use a potato masher or an immersion blender to mash the vegetables. For a smooth puree, blend the mixture in a food processor, and then return to the saucepan and reheat. Transfer to a bowl and garnish with chives before serving.

Creamy Vegetables "Alfredo"

Serves 4

A light and creamy sauce with some aromatic garlic is spooned over cooked vegetables. Could not be more delicious or easy to make. If you use this as a side dish, keep the main course simple, too—a steak, a burger, or some grilled fish.

1 can full-fat coconut milk, divided

3 cloves garlic, minced

1 teaspoon fine sea salt

½ teaspoon freshly ground
    black pepper

1 tablespoon tapioca flour

4 cups cooked vegetables of your
    choice (broccoli, cauliflower,
    spinach, etc.)

Measure out ¼ cup coconut milk and put aside.

In a saucepan, simmer the rest of the coconut milk, garlic, salt, and pepper for 5 minutes.

In a separate bowl, whisk together the tapioca flour and the ¼ cup coconut milk. Add to the saucepan and stir until thickened. Serve over cooked vegetables.

Loaded and Baked Sweet Potatoes

Serves 4

These are a big hit in our house. We buy sweet potatoes by the dozens and use them in so many ways. You can load baked sweet potatoes with just about anything—Bison Chili (page 164), Wilted Greens with Bacon (page 193), or Spinach-Artichoke Dip (page 223), to name a few.

2 sweet potatoes

2 slices pastured and
    nitrate-free bacon

½ onion, chopped

1 clove garlic, minced

½ teaspoon freshly ground
    black pepper

¼ teaspoon fine sea salt

Heat oven to 450°F. Line a sheet pan with parchment paper.

Pierce the sweet potatoes all over with a fork and place them on the prepared sheet pan. Bake for 50 minutes, or until tender and can be pierced with a knife. Keep the oven on.

While the sweet potatoes are cooking, heat a skillet over medium-high heat. Add the bacon and cook until crisp, turning as necessary. Put the cooked bacon on paper towels to drain. When cool enough to handle, chop the bacon and put in a bowl. Add the onion and garlic to the hot skillet and sauté for 5 minutes, then add to the bacon.

When the sweet potatoes are done and cool enough to handle, slice them in half horizontally. Scrape out the flesh with a spoon. Add the flesh to the bacon mixture. Season with salt and pepper and mix. Spoon the sweet potato mixture into the four skins. Arrange on the prepared pan. Bake for 20 to 25 minutes, until lightly brown on top.

Broccolini with Garlic and Lemon

Serves 2

Like mother, like daughter. Elle loves my favorite vegetable as much as I do. Broccolini has smaller florets and longer stems than broccoli, so there's no need to cut it up. You can also roast broccolini, tossed with a little olive oil, in a 400°F oven. Both methods work as well with cauliflower, asparagus, brussels sprouts, and dark, leafy greens.

1 bunch broccolini (about ½ pound)

1 tablespoon avocado oil

3 garlic cloves, thinly sliced

½ lemon

Place a steamer basket in a large saucepan. Add 2 inches water. Arrange the broccolini in the basket. Cover, turn on the heat to high, and steam until tender, but not too soft, about 5 minutes.

Heat the oil and garlic in a skillet over medium heat. Sauté until fragrant, about 1 minute, taking care not to burn the garlic. Add the broccolini to the pan and cook for 5 minutes, tossing regularly. Squeeze lemon juice over the broccolini before serving.

Wilted Greens with Bacon

Serves 2

Having grown up in the South, it would be improper for me to write a cookbook and not include a recipe for wilted greens. Cooked greens are a staple food where I come from. Kale, swiss chard, arugula, spinach, watercress, and collard, turnip, and mustard greens can be cooked individually or in combinations. If you don't have any bacon fat on hand, cook two strips in a skillet and use the rendered fat to sauté the greens. Then crumble bacon pieces on top of the greens. The bacon makes all the difference in this dish.

1 clove garlic, minced

1 tablespoon bacon fat

4 packed cups trimmed and cut-up greens

In a skillet over medium-high heat, sauté the garlic in the bacon fat for 1 to 2 minutes. Add the greens and sauté until lightly wilted and coated. Crumble bacon pieces on top of the greens. Serve.

Grilled Bok Choy

Bok choy is a versatile vegetable in the Chinese cabbage family that can be sautéed, roasted, or grilled. Serve with grilled shrimp or fish and some Cauliflower Rice (page 67).

Serves 4

½ cup Gut-Healing Bone Broth
(page 71)

2 teaspoons fish sauce

2 teaspoons coconut aminos

2 teaspoons honey

1 pound baby bok choy, sliced in
half through the root end

Heat a grill pan or an outdoor grill.

In a bowl, whisk together the broth, fish sauce, coconut aminos, and honey. Add the bok choy and gently toss to coat. Cook 2 to 3 minutes on all sides, until slightly wilted.

9

Dressings, Sauces, and Condiments

You're going to love making the switch to these autoimmune-friendly, real-food versions of your favorite flavorful dressings, sauces, and condiments! Toss Spinach-Kale Pesto (page 196) with your spiralized veggie noodles for a taste of Tuscany, dip your veggies in garlicky Aïoli (page 197) for a Mediterranean-inspired snack, or add tomato-free No-Mato Sauce (page 198) to your burgers for an American classic.

Once you see how easy it is to make your own delectable dressings, sauces, and condiments, you'll be so glad you ditched the packaged versions with their hidden sugars and gluten, artificial ingredients, and toxic chemicals!

Spinach-Kale Pesto

Makes 1½ cups

Pesto was a staple in our house when I was growing up. We had a large herb garden, and I used to help my mom pick the fresh basil. The pesto I make now is a bit different from when I was a kid, but I make a jar of it at least once a week in the spring and keep it in my fridge. Toss with spiralized vegetable noodles. Load some onto a baked sweet potato or butternut squash. Use it with the Chicken Rollatini with Bacon and Pesto (page 154) and Pesto Pizza (page 166). It's a great condiment with burgers, steaks, shrimp, or fish and also a tasty vegetable dip. This pesto is a powerful source of selenium and zinc, which are important for a healthy immune system and thyroid.

4 cups loosely packed spinach

2 cups chopped kale leaves

12 cloves garlic, peeled and
    smashed

2 handfuls basil leaves

1 teaspoon fine sea salt

½ cup freshly squeezed lemon juice

½ cup extra virgin olive oil

Combine the spinach, kale, garlic, basil, salt, and lemon juice in a food processor or high-speed blender. Process or blend just until the greens are chopped.

With the motor running, slowly drizzle half of the olive oil through the feed tube of the food processor or top of the blender. The pesto should be creamy and entirely smooth. Stop the machine and scrape down the sides with a spatula. Add the remaining olive oil through the top and pulse until combined. Store in the refrigerator up to 1 week or in the freezer for 2 months. If frozen, thaw before using.

Aïoli

Aïoli is a garlicky, mayonnaise-like Mediterranean sauce. Spoon this eggless version over fish, shrimp, and cooked vegetables or use it as a dip.

3 to 4 cloves garlic, roasted (page 73)

¼ cup palm shortening

⅓ cup avocado oil

2 teaspoons apple cider vinegar

½ teaspoon fine sea salt

Put all ingredients into a food processor or blender and process until combined. Refrigerate in a glass jar for up to 2 weeks.

No-Mato Sauce

Makes 1 cup

Pour this rich puree of carrots, beets, and seasoning over vegetable noodles and add to soups for another layer of flavor. Tomatoes aren't included because they're a member of the nightshade family and may contribute to inflammation.

1 tablespoon avocado oil

3 cloves garlic, minced

½ onion, finely chopped

2 carrots, chopped

1 small beet, peeled and cut
  into quarters

2 tablespoons Gut-Healing Bone
  Broth (page 71)

½ cup basil leaves

1 tablespoon apple cider vinegar

1 teaspoon fine sea salt

¼ cup extra virgin olive oil

Heat the oil in a skillet over medium-high heat. Add the garlic and onions and sauté until fragrant. Set aside.

In a saucepan, add the carrots to 1 cup water. Bring to a boil, then lower the heat to a simmer and cook 4 to 6 minutes, or until carrots are fork tender. Remove carrots from water and set aside. Add beets to the water. Bring to a boil, then lower the heat to a simmer and cook for 4 to 6 minutes. The water should begin turning red from the beets. Remove beets from the water and save them for later use with another recipe or meal. Reserve the cooking water.

Place the garlic, onion, 4 tablespoons of beet water, and all remaining ingredients except for olive oil into a food processor or high-speed blender. Puree until a sauce is formed. While food processor or blender is running, drizzle in olive oil and blend until smooth.

Ketchup

Makes 2 cups

What's a burger and fries without ketchup? Here's my version of this popular condiment. Enjoy it with The Perfect Fast Man Burgers (page 162), Sweet Potato Fries (page 185), or Spaghetti Squash Hash Browns (page 91).

1 tablespoon avocado oil

½ onion, chopped

2 carrots, chopped

1 small beet, chopped and
    quartered

2 tablespoons apple cider vinegar

2 tablespoons freshly squeezed
    lemon juice

½ tablespoon garlic powder

1 teaspoon onion powder

2 tablespoons honey

1 teaspoon fine sea salt

Heat oil in a skillet to medium-high heat. Add the onions and sauté until translucent. Set aside.

In a saucepan, add the carrots to 1 cup water. Bring to a boil, then lower the heat to a simmer and cook 4 to 6 minutes, or until carrots are fork tender. Remove carrots from water and set aside. Add beets to the water. Bring to a boil, then lower the heat to a simmer and cook for 4 to 6 minutes. The water should begin turning red from the beets. Remove beets from water and save them for later use with another recipe or meal. Reserve the cooking water.

Add the onion, 3 tablespoons of beet water, and all remaining ingredients to a food processor or high-speed blender. Puree until sauce is formed. Place in refrigerator and let cool.

Cherry Barbecue Sauce

Makes 1 cup

Brush this sweet-and-sour sauce over lamb, pork chops, or chicken before grilling. Keep an extra bowl of the sauce on the table for dipping. This recipe works wonderfully on Braised Pork Ribs (page 171).

4 carrots, chopped

½ cup pitted fresh or frozen
   sweet cherries

½ onion, finely chopped

¼ cup Gut-Healing Bone Broth
   (page 71)

2 tablespoons molasses

2 tablespoons maple syrup

1 tablespoon freshly squeezed
   lemon juice

1 tablespoon apple cider vinegar

¼ teaspoon freshly ground
   black pepper

½ teaspoon fine sea salt

In a saucepan, add the carrots to 1 cup water. Bring to a boil, then lower the heat to a simmer and cook 4 to 6 minutes, or until carrots are fork tender. Drain carrots.

In the saucepan over medium-high heat, add the cherries, onion, and broth. Bring to a boil, then lower the heat to a simmer. Add the remaining ingredients and cook on medium-low heat for 20 to 25 minutes, stirring occasionally. Transfer mixture to a food processor or high-speed blender. Blend until combined, and store in the refrigerator.

"Peanut" Sauce

Makes 1 cup

Here's my take on Asian peanut sauce. It has a "nutty" flavor and creamy texture. It's perfect with Chicken Pad Thai (page 156), Chicken Satay with "Peanut" Sauce (page 226), and grilled shrimp.

½ cup Tigernut Butter (page 219)

¼ cup Gut-Healing Bone Broth (page 71)

1 tablespoon apple cider vinegar

½ tablespoon honey

½ tablespoon coconut aminos

½-inch piece of fresh ginger, peeled

Place all ingredients in a food processor or high-speed blender.

Blend until smooth, but thick.

Refrigerate in a glass jar up to 1 week.

Meat Marinade

Makes 1 cup, enough for 1 to 2 pounds of meat

One of Xavier's favorite pastimes is grilling. He uses this marinade on vegetables, steaks, burgers, chicken, and fish. It's particularly wonderful with the Carolina Pulled Pork (page 169).

2 cloves garlic, minced

4 teaspoons onion powder

½ cup coconut aminos

2 teaspoons freshly ground
black pepper

3 tablespoons honey

½ cup Gut-Healing Bone Broth
(page 71)

In a shallow dish, large enough to hold the meat in a single layer, whisk together all of the ingredients.

Add the meat to the marinade and refrigerate from 1 to 24 hours, turning every so often.

Bring the meat to room temperature before grilling. Discard any leftover marinade.

The World's Best Asian Marinade

Makes about 1 cup, enough for 1 to 2 pounds of meat

I already mentioned that Xavier and I used this marinade on the beef tenderloins we served at our wedding. The toasted sesame oil in this recipe adds an Asian touch. Use this marinade for the World's Best Asian Flank Steak (page 161). It's also great for skewers of vegetables, shrimp, or chicken.

½ cup coconut aminos

½ cup toasted sesame oil

2 tablespoons honey

2 garlic cloves, minced

2 tablespoons fish sauce

1 tablespoon grated fresh ginger

In a shallow dish, large enough to hold the meat in a single layer, whisk together all of the ingredients.

Add the meat to the marinade and refrigerate from 1 to 24 hours, turning every so often.

Bring the meat to room temperature before grilling. Discard any leftover marinade.

Tzatziki

This is a dairy-free version of the classic Greek herbed yogurt. It is generally served chilled and can be used as a sauce on top of grilled meats or vegetables. As a dip, pair it with Root Vegetable Chips (page 215) or raw vegetables.

½ cup Coconut Milk Yogurt
   (page 70)

½ cucumber, peeled and grated

2 tablespoons freshly squeezed
   lemon juice

1 tablespoon apple cider vinegar

1 clove garlic, minced

¾ teaspoon fine sea salt

¾ teaspoon freshly ground
   black pepper

¼ teaspoon fresh dill

Whisk together all of the ingredients in a bowl. Use immediately or cover and refrigerate up to 1 week.

Betty's Italian Dressing

Makes about 2 cups

I already mentioned that my mom was famous for her amazing salads and that we had a large bowl of salad on the dinner table every night when I was growing up. Though she is no longer with us, I am pleased to share her delicious Italian dressing with each of you.

1 cup extra virgin olive oil

4 cloves garlic, minced

½ teaspoon onion powder

½ teaspoon ground ginger

1 tablespoon raw honey

1 tablespoon Dijon mustard

½ cup apple cider vinegar

½ teaspoon fine sea salt

½ teaspoon freshly ground
  black pepper

Put all ingredients in a medium bowl and whisk together. Store dressing in a sealed glass jar at room temperature. If ingredients separate during storage, shake to combine before use.

Ranch Dressing

Makes about 2 cups

Drizzle this Ranch Dressing on salads and cooked vegetables. Spread some on burgers or even baked sweet potatoes. Coconut milk is used instead of the processed buttermilk and mayonnaise usually found in this dressing.

1 tablespoon fresh parsley

1 tablespoon garlic powder

1 tablespoon onion powder

2 teaspoons dried dill

1 teaspoon fine sea salt

½ teaspoon freshly ground black pepper

2 cups full-fat coconut milk

3 tablespoons apple cider vinegar

Mix the parsley, garlic powder, onion powder, dill, salt, and pepper in a bowl.

In a separate bowl, whisk together the coconut milk and vinegar. Whisk the seasoning mix into the coconut milk–vinegar mixture, stirring well to combine. Serve immediately or cover and refrigerate for up to 2 weeks.

Blackberry Vinaigrette

Makes 1 cup

When I was a child, my family moved to the Mississippi Gulf Coast for a year. We had wonderful times picking blackberries along the train tracks. My dad and I made blackberry jam, and my mom made a vinaigrette similar to this one. Toss this dressing with a salad of leftover steak, spinach, and red onion. Blackberry season is short, so feel free to use frozen ones in the recipe.

2 cups fresh or frozen and thawed blackberries

1 teaspoon honey

1 teaspoon fresh thyme leaves

2 tablespoons apple cider vinegar

½ cup extra virgin olive oil

½ teaspoon fine sea salt

In a food processor or high-speed blender, combine all ingredients and puree. Use immediately or refrigerate in a glass jar for up to 1 week.

Herbed Vinaigrette

Makes 1 cup

The powerfully flavorful combination of herbs in this dressing will please even the most demanding gourmet. Feel free to add in or substitute dill, parsley, mint, basil, or oregano.

¾ cup extra virgin olive oil

¼ cup apple cider vinegar

1 teaspoon freshly squeezed
   lemon juice

1 teaspoon fresh thyme leaves

1 teaspoon fresh tarragon leaves

1 shallot, finely chopped

Pinch fine sea salt

Pinch freshly ground black pepper

Whisk together all ingredients. If ingredients separate during storage, shake to combine before use. Store at room temperature.

Green Goddess Dressing

Makes 1 cup

This is an AmyMyersMD.com team favorite and is always on the table at team meetings and potlucks. This dressing is so versatile, you can use it as a dressing, sauce, or a dip.

½ cup chopped fresh parsley

¼ cup chopped fresh tarragon

3 tablespoons chopped fresh chives

1 clove garlic

1 avocado, peeled and pitted

2 tablespoons fresh lemon juice

3 tablespoons extra virgin olive oil

Place all ingredients in a high-speed blender or food processor and puree. Cover and refrigerate in a covered glass container for up to 5 days.

Mango-Avocado Salsa

Makes 2 cups

For a dip, serve with BLC Tacos (page 88) or Plantain Chips (page 216), or use as the salsa for grilled fish, shrimp, or chicken. Roll some up in lettuce leaves for an appetizer or snack.

1 mango, cubed

1 avocado, cubed

½ red onion, finely chopped

3 tablespoons chopped
   fresh cilantro

Juice of 1 small lime

1 tablespoon extra virgin olive oil

¼ teaspoon fine sea salt

½ teaspoon freshly ground
   black pepper

½ teaspoon ground cumin

In a bowl, combine all ingredients and mix gently. Serve immediately.

Fruit Compotes

Serves 2

These chunky fruit compotes are wonderful with a trickle of syrup on Tigernut Waffles (page 95) or Pumpkin Pancakes (page 96).

Apple-Cinnamon Compote

1 tablespoon coconut oil

½ apple, cored and sliced

½ teaspoon ground cinnamon

¼ teaspoon ground nutmeg

In a saucepan, heat the coconut oil over medium-low heat. Stir in the apples, cinnamon, and nutmeg. Cook until the apples are fork tender and cooked through, about 5 minutes.

Blueberry-Lemon Compote

1 tablespoon coconut oil

2 cups fresh or frozen blueberries

Zest of ½ lemon

In a saucepan, heat the coconut oil over medium-low heat. Stir in the blueberries and lemon zest. Cook until the blueberries are soft and sauce-like, about 5 minutes.

Caramelized Banana Compote

1 tablespoon coconut oil

1 banana, sliced

1 tablespoon maple syrup

½ teaspoon ground cinnamon

In a saucepan, heat the coconut oil over medium-low heat. Add the banana, maple syrup, and cinnamon. Cook until the bananas are soft and lightly browned, about 5 minutes.

Tapenade

This olive spread from the South of France is a perfect appetizer when accompanied by endive leaves, celery, or fennel. A spoonful or two goes well with grilled fish or chicken. Use a variety of olives for color and flavor. The secret is not to overprocess the tapenade. It should be coarse, not smooth.

⅓ cup pitted green olives

⅓ cup pitted black olives

⅓ cup pitted Kalamata olives

1 clove garlic

1 teaspoon capers, rinsed and drained

1 teaspoon apple cider vinegar

2 tablespoons extra virgin olive oil

In a food processor, combine the olives, garlic, capers, and vinegar. Pulse until coarsely chopped and well blended. Continue to process, slowly adding the olive oil through the feed tube.

Serve at room temperature. Refrigerate for up to 1 week.

10

Snacks

"Be Prepared" isn't just the Boy Scout motto! It's my motto for maintaining The Myers Way, too, and it's super easy to be prepared with these tasty snacks that are rich in immune-boosting and gut-healing nutrients.

You will find plenty of options in this chapter to give you a burst of energy, satisfy your hunger cravings, and fuel your brain—all while keeping you on track with The Myers Way. I recommend preparing snacks in advance so you always have them on hand. That way, next time you're stuck in a meeting or caught in traffic and hunger strikes, you can simply reach for a handful of Sweet-and-Salty Trail Mix (page 214), Coconut Collagen Fuel Bites (page 218), or Rosemary–Sea Salt Crackers (page 222).

And don't keep all of these delicious treats to yourself—children will love them too!

Sweet-and-Salty Trail Mix

Makes 8 cups

I travel at least once a month, and it's hard to find The Myers Way–approved foods in airports or on the road. This trail mix has been a lifesaver for me and my family. Before any trip, I whip up a batch and take it with me. Be sure to purchase no-sugar-added and sulfate-free dried fruit.

1 cup whole tigernuts

2 cups unsweetened coconut flakes

2 cups chopped and mixed dried
    fruit, such as cranberries,
    cherries, blueberries, and apple

1 cup Plantain Chips (page 216)

1 cup Root Vegetable Chips
    (page 215)

Soak the tigernuts in cool water, just enough to cover, overnight. Drain the water. Lay tigernuts flat on a towel to dry.

Heat oven to 325°F. Line a sheet pan with parchment paper.

Spread the coconut flakes onto the prepared pan. Watching carefully so the coconut doesn't burn, toast for 3 to 5 minutes, tossing once to brown evenly. When lightly browned, remove from the oven and let cool.

In a bowl, toss the coconut with the remaining ingredients. Store in a glass container at room temperature.

Root Vegetable Chips

Serves 4

Homemade vegetable chips go in Sweet-and-Salty Trail Mix (page 214) and can be dipped into Spinach-Artichoke Dip (page 223) and Tzatziki (page 204)—or any other dips in this book. Here's another recipe where your mandoline comes in handy for making paper-thin vegetable slices. The instructions below say to store these chips in a glass jar at room temperature, but trust me, they won't last very long!

1 medium sweet potato, peeled and sliced 1/16 inch thick

1 small golden beet, peeled and sliced 1/16 inch thick

2 large carrots, peeled and sliced 1/16 inch thick

2 large parsnips, peeled and sliced 1/16 inch thick

1 medium turnip, peeled and sliced 1/16 inch thick

2 teaspoons fine sea salt

3 tablespoons avocado oil

Optional Seasonings: Garlic powder, dried rosemary, freshly ground black pepper, cinnamon, onion powder

Heat oven to 400°F. Line two sheet pans with parchment paper.

Put the sliced vegetables in a colander and sprinkle them with salt. Let the vegetables sit for 15 minutes.

Arrange the vegetable slices between cloth or paper towels and press out as much excess water as possible.

Put the vegetables in a bowl and toss thoroughly with the avocado oil. Arrange the vegetables in a single layer on the prepared sheet pans. Sprinkle with your choice of spices. Bake for 20 to 25 minutes, until crispy. Let cool on paper towels before storing in a glass container at room temperature.

Plantain Chips

Serves 2

When it's vacation time, Xavier and I like to escape to Nicaragua where the sand is white, the ocean is clear blue, and the food is fresh, clean, and delicious. It's a treat to sit in lounge chairs under umbrellas and scoop fresh guacamole with freshly made plantain chips. Even when plantains are ripe, they're hard and need to be cooked. These plantain chips go well with Mango-Avocado Salsa (page 210), Tropical Nicaraguan Salad (page 144), or Five-Vegetable Guacamole (page 220).

2 plantains, peeled and sliced $\frac{1}{16}$ inch thick

$\frac{1}{4}$ cup coconut oil, melted

Optional Seasonings: Sea salt, freshly ground black pepper, garlic powder, onion powder, cinnamon

Heat oven to 350°F. Line a sheet pan with parchment paper.

Put the sliced plantains in a bowl and toss with coconut oil to coat evenly.

Arrange the plantain slices in a single layer on the prepared pan and season with desired seasonings. Bake for 20 to 25 minutes, until brown on the edges. Keep an eye on the chips to prevent them from burning. Store in a glass jar at room temperature.

Rutabaga "Hummus"

Makes 1½ cups

Rutabagas, a root vegetable often called "yellow turnips," don't get the attention they deserve. They are rich in fiber, vitamin C, and minerals like potassium and manganese. Best when mashed, they can be combined with carrots and sweet potatoes or used in this spread. Serve with fresh vegetables and Rosemary–Sea Salt Crackers (page 222).

2 cups chopped rutabaga	1 teaspoon ground cumin
Juice of ½ large lemon	½ teaspoon fine sea salt
1 clove garlic, roasted (page 73)	¼ cup extra virgin olive oil

Place rutabaga pieces in a saucepan and cover with water. Bring to a boil; then lower the heat to a simmer and cook until the pieces can be pierced easily with a knife, about 10 minutes. Drain the rutabaga in a colander and let cool.

Place the rutabaga, lemon juice, garlic, cumin, and salt in a food processor and pulse. Stop the machine and scrape the sides. Slowly add the olive oil through the feed tube and pulse to puree. Serve at room temperature or refrigerate in a glass container for 1 to 2 weeks.

Coconut Collagen Fuel Bites

Makes 12 bites

These are great to eat after a workout, while on a hike, when traveling, or as a sweet treat for dessert. The combination of healthy fats from the coconut oil and coconut butter and protein-rich collagen will keep you satisfied for hours without wrecking your metabolism.

½ cup coconut oil

½ cup coconut butter

2 scoops The Myers Way Collagen
 Protein (or similar collagen)

¼ teaspoon powdered stevia

3 drops peppermint oil *or*

 2 teaspoons freshly squeezed
 lemon juice

Put the coconut oil and coconut butter into a saucepan over medium heat to melt.

Remove the pan from the heat and stir in the collagen, stevia, and flavoring of your choice.

Pour the mixture carefully into a parchment-lined 8-by-8-inch baking dish or nonstick silicone candy molds.

Place in the refrigerator and let sit until hardened.

Cut into bites or carefully pop out of molds.

Tigernut Butter

Makes 1 cup

Looking for an alternative to peanut or almond butter? Meet tigernut butter! Tigernuts are soaked in water and then pureed with coconut oil and a little sweetener to make a spread that you can enjoy on apple slices or Zucchini Muffins (page 97). Tigernuts are loaded with prebiotic fiber to feed the good bacteria in your gut.

½ cup whole tigernuts

2 tablespoons coconut oil

1 teaspoon maple syrup

Soak tigernuts in water for 1 hour or overnight.

Place tigernuts in a food processor or high-speed blender. Blend for 1 minute.

Scrape down sides and add the coconut oil and maple syrup. Blend until combined. Store in a glass container in the refrigerator for 1 to 2 weeks.

Five-Vegetable Guacamole

Serves 4

You'll find endless ways to enjoy this variation of an all-time favorite. Enjoy solo with a spoon or pair some with burgers, kebobs, chicken, or fish. Serve with kale chips or Plantain Chips (page 216). Pair it with BLC Tacos (page 88) or a Chicken Burrito Bowl (page 157).

2 avocados, peeled, pitted, and mashed

½ onion, diced

½ cucumber, julienned

½ yellow squash, grated

½ zucchini, grated

2 carrots, julienned

1 clove garlic, minced

Juice from ½ lime

2 tablespoons chopped cilantro

Fine sea salt, to taste

Lime wedges

Combine all ingredients except the sea salt and lime wedges in a bowl. Season with salt to taste.

Serve immediately or cover and refrigerate for 1 to 2 days. Serve with lime wedges.

Fruit Snacks

Makes 9 gummies

Kids and adults love these healthy snack alternatives to gummy bears and processed fruit gummies. Nonstick silicone candy molds come in all sizes and shapes—stars, hearts, animals—and can be purchased at craft stores, supermarkets, and online. If you don't have silicone candy molds, pour the mixture into an 8-by-8-inch baking dish. Chill until firm and then use small cookie cutters to cut out desired shapes.

½ cup unsweetened pomegranate juice

2 tablespoons The Myers Way Gelatin (or similar gelatin)

1 teaspoon powdered stevia

To a small saucepan, add the juice, gelatin, and stevia. Whisk to combine and let sit for about 5 minutes so the gelatin "blooms."

Place saucepan over low-medium heat. As the mixture heats up, it will start to liquefy. Once the gelatin is dissolved, turn off the heat. Whisk once or twice to combine.

Pour the mixture carefully into a parchment-lined sheet pan for "fruit leather" or into silicone molds for "gummies."

Refrigerate the pan or molds for about 2 hours or until fully set. Then cut into "fruit leather" strips, or carefully pop gummies out of molds and place in a storage container in the fridge.

Apple Snacks: Replace the pomegranate juice with ½ cup 100 percent apple juice.

Raspberry-Lemon Snacks: Replace the pomegranate juice with ½ cup raspberries pureed with 1 tablespoon freshly squeezed lemon juice.

Mixed Berry Snacks: Replace the pomegranate juice with ½ cup mixed and pureed berries, such as blackberries, raspberries, blueberries, and strawberries.

Rosemary-Sea Salt Crackers

Finally, a real cracker that we can eat! Dip in Rutabaga "Hummus" (page 217), Spinach-Artichoke Dip (page 223), or Five-Vegetable Guacamole (page 220). You can use dried thyme, dill, oregano, or fennel seeds in combination with the rosemary or alone in these crisp crackers. Make two batches, because believe me, they won't last long!

Makes 10 to 12 crackers

1 cup cassava flour

1 teaspoon aluminum-free
  baking powder

1 teaspoon fine sea salt

½ cup filtered water

2 tablespoons extra virgin olive oil,
  plus extra for brushing on dough

Sea salt flakes, to taste

½ tablespoon chopped fresh
  rosemary leaves

Heat oven to 400°F. In a mixing bowl, combine the cassava flour, baking powder, and sea salt. Mix in water and olive oil. Stir until the ingredients come together.

Turn the dough out onto parchment paper lightly dusted with cassava flour. Using a rolling pin, roll the dough about 1/16 to 1/8 inch thick. Brush the dough with olive oil. Sprinkle on the sea salt and rosemary and lightly press into the dough. Using a knife, slice dough into squares. Transfer the parchment paper to a sheet pan.

Bake for 20 minutes or until golden brown. Let cool on a wire rack. Store the crackers in an airtight container.

Spinach-Artichoke Dip

Serves 6 to 8

Growing up, I looked forward to my aunt's famous spinach-artichoke dip every Christmas. She made her dip with cheese and mayonnaise, but here's The Myers Way–approved adaptation. Serve this party dip with Plantain Chips (page 216), Sweet Potato Fries (page 185), Rosemary–Sea Salt Crackers (page 222), or Belgian endive leaves.

1 14-ounce can artichoke hearts, drained and coarsely chopped

1 tablespoon avocado oil

½ onion, chopped

1 clove garlic, minced

1 cup frozen or 2 cups fresh spinach

1 15-ounce can coconut cream

2 tablespoons Aïoli (page 197)

1 tablespoon freshly squeezed lemon juice

¼ teaspoon fine sea salt

Heat oven to 400°F. In a skillet, sauté the garlic and onion in the avocado oil until fragrant, about 2 minutes. Add the spinach and artichoke hearts and sauté until the spinach is wilted. Transfer to a bowl and stir in the coconut cream, aïoli, lemon juice, and salt.

Evenly spread the mixture into an 8-by-8-inch baking dish and bake for 30 minutes. Serve warm.

Beef Jerky

Homemade beef jerky is a go-to snack for me and my family, especially when we're traveling. It's easy to pack and doesn't require refrigeration. Many of the commercial brands are made from beef that's not grass-fed and pasture-raised or they contain unwanted ingredients, such as soy sauce or sugar. When butterflying steak, chicken breast, or fish, cut the meat horizontally into two even pieces—but not all the way. The two pieces will be "bound" together on one side like a book, and then when you cook the meat, you "open" it like a book—or butterfly wings. You can use thinly sliced top round or eye of round in place of flank steak.

1 pound 100 percent grass-fed and pasture-raised flank steak

Meat Marinade (page 202) *or* The World's Best Asian Marinade (page 203)

Lay the flank steak flat on a cutting board. Use a sharp knife to butterfly the steak; place your other hand flat on top of the steak to hold it secure as you cut, keeping the knife level with the cutting board.

Open the meat, like a book. With a meat mallet, pound the steak to ⅛- to ¼-inch thickness. Place in a shallow dish. Pour the marinade over the meat and marinate for 30 minutes or overnight.

Heat oven to 175°F. Line a sheet pan with parchment paper and place it on the bottom rack of the oven. Place meat on a removable wire rack placed on top of the sheet pan or directly on the top oven rack to allow for air circulation around the meat. Bake for 5 hours or until dried and cooked through. Remove and let cool completely before storing in a glass container in the refrigerator.

Wild-Caught Shrimp Sushi Rolls

Serves 6

This is a favorite from The Thyroid Connection. *Kids love to make hand rolls! Nori, a flat seaweed, is easy to find and provides an excellent source of iodine, which the body needs to make thyroid hormones. You can omit the shrimp, if you wish, or add sushi-grade, wild-caught salmon, blanched asparagus, or roasted cubes of sweet potato or butternut squash. A platter of sushi rolls makes a stunning appetizer.*

6 sheets nori

1 large avocado, mashed

1 tablespoon fresh ginger, peeled and grated

1 packed cup baby spinach leaves

18 wild-caught shrimp (16–20 count), cooked and deveined

⅓ cup thinly cut carrots, like matchsticks

1 cucumber, thinly sliced

2 lemon wedges

Place 1 nori sheet on a cutting board. Using a spatula, spread a thin layer of avocado over the entire surface of the nori. Sprinkle some grated ginger on top of the avocado, followed by some spinach. Place a row of shrimp along the bottom edge of the avocado-covered nori sheet, followed by a row of carrots on top of the shrimp, and then a row of cucumbers.

Starting from the bottom, fold the nori over all the ingredients, then roll tightly until compact. Slice into individual rolls.

Repeat the steps with the remaining ingredients. Put the rolls on a platter and serve with the lemon wedges.

Chicken Satay with "Peanut" Sauce

Serves 8

Indonesian satay is a dish of skewered pieces of chicken or other meats that are brushed with a sauce and then grilled. You can find wooden skewers in any supermarket. Be sure to soak the skewers in water before using so they don't burn. Accompany with Cauliflower Rice (page 67), Vegetable Fried "Rice" (page 177), or Chicken Pad Thai (page 156) for a main course or serve them as an appetizer at your next party.

8 wooden skewers

1 2-inch piece of lemongrass, outer leaves removed and finely chopped

2 cloves garlic, minced

2 tablespoons coconut aminos

1 teaspoon fish sauce

1 teaspoon honey

Juice of 1 lime

1 tablespoon avocado oil

1 pound free-range skinless, boneless chicken breasts, sliced into 1-inch pieces

"Peanut" Sauce (page 201)

Soak the skewers in water for 30 minutes.

In a bowl, whisk together the lemongrass, garlic, coconut aminos, fish sauce, honey, and lime juice. Thread the chicken pieces onto the soaked skewers. Brush the sauce onto the chicken, making sure to cover well.

Brush the avocado oil on a grill pan and heat over high. Grill the chicken skewers for 3 to 5 minutes on each side, brushing with more sauce halfway through. Remove the skewers from the pan and serve with "Peanut" Sauce.

11

Desserts

Dessert lovers (myself included), rejoice! With new options such as cassava, arrowroot, and coconut flours; coconut sugar; gelatin; and other approved ingredients, you can indulge in a slice of pie, a cookie, or chocolate mousse on special occasions while still supporting your health! Just remember that if you have Candida overgrowth or SIBO (visit amymd.io/quiz to find out), I recommend holding off on any form of sugar until those infections have been eliminated.

More good news: the recipes in this chapter use fewer ingredients and simpler techniques than traditional baked treats or sweets, so they're easier to make—and just as easy to enjoy!

In this chapter you'll find autoimmune-friendly versions of classics such as brownies, cupcakes, lemon bars, gingerbread, and pumpkin pie, as well as decadent new treats to try for the first time. Whether you're celebrating at home or taking dessert to a party, you can serve a sweet treat that everyone will love!

Anne's Amazing Cinnamon-Raisin Cookies

Makes 9 cookies

I received these cookies as a birthday gift from the wife (Anne) of one of my team members. They remind me so much of the oatmeal raisin cookies my mom used to bake and that I haven't been able to enjoy since following The Myers Way. These cookies are perfectly fluffy on the inside and delightfully crisp on the outside. A light splash of cinnamon along with the sweet flavor of raisins make these cookies feel nostalgic, while still being 100 percent The Myers Way–compliant. In fact, I requested these for Christmas from my Secret Santa this year. Anne was kind enough to let me share this recipe with all of you—thank you, Anne!

¼ cup palm shortening

2 tablespoons pure maple syrup

¼ cup coconut sugar

1½ teaspoons pure vanilla extract

¾ cup arrowroot flour

¼ cup tigernut flour

1 tablespoon The Myers Way Gelatin (or similar gelatin)

1 teaspoon aluminum-free baking soda

½ teaspoon cream of tartar

2 teaspoons ground cinnamon

½ teaspoon fine sea salt

¼ cup raisins

Heat oven to 350°F. Grease a baking sheet pan with either coconut oil or palm shortening.

In the large bowl of an electric mixer, add the palm shortening, maple syrup, sugar, and vanilla. Beat until creamy.

In another bowl, whisk together the arrowroot flour, tigernut flour, gelatin, baking soda, cream of tartar, cinnamon, and sea salt.

Slowly add dry ingredients to the wet ingredients and beat on medium to combine. Using a spatula, fold in the raisins. Note: This yields a dry and crumbly dough, but it will form into balls easily. If your dough will not stick together, add another tablespoon of palm shortening for more moisture.

Using clean hands, form pieces of the dough into 1-inch balls. Place balls 2 inches apart on the prepared pan. Bake for 10 to 12 minutes.

Remove pan from oven and let cookies cool on the pan for 5 to 10 minutes before moving them to a rack to cool completely.

Gingerbread Cake

Serves 8

My mom made gingerbread cake and gingerbread cookies from scratch when I was growing up. I am so excited to present you with this autoimmune-friendly version of my mom's famous gingerbread cake! Gingerbread is all about the fragrant spices, so make sure yours are fresh.

Cake

1 cup cassava flour

⅔ cup coconut flour

⅓ cup arrowroot flour

1 tablespoon The Myers Way Gelatin (or similar gelatin)

2 teaspoons baking soda

2 teaspoons ground cinnamon

2 teaspoons ground ginger

1 teaspoon ground cardamom

1 teaspoon ground allspice

½ teaspoon ground cloves

½ teaspoon cream of tartar

½ teaspoon fine sea salt

1 cup unsweetened applesauce

¾ cup filtered water

¼ cup coconut oil

⅓ cup maple syrup

1 tablespoon pure vanilla extract

Glaze

¼ cup coconut butter

2 tablespoons maple syrup

2 tablespoons filtered water or coconut milk

Heat oven to 350°F. Grease an 8-by-4-inch loaf pan with melted coconut oil.

To make the cake: In the bowl of an electric mixer, combine the cassava flour, coconut flour, arrowroot flour, gelatin, baking soda, cinnamon, ginger, cardamom, allspice, cloves, cream of tartar, and sea salt. On low speed, mix the dry ingredients together.

Add the applesauce, water, coconut oil, maple syrup, and vanilla to the dry ingredients and mix at medium speed for 1 to 2 minutes. The batter will be thick.

Pour in the prepared pan and bake for 50 minutes, until a toothpick in the center comes out clean.

To make the glaze: In a saucepan, combine the coconut butter, maple syrup, and water over low heat until a glaze forms. Whisk together and set aside.

Remove cake from the oven and let cool completely before turning out of the pan. Pour glaze on top and slice to serve.

Fudgy Brownies

Makes 8 brownies

What's better than biting into a smooth, rich, chocolaty, fudgy brownie? Add Coconut Chocolate Mousse (page 245) or its vanilla cinnamon option for à la mode. These are perfect for school bake sales and treat days.

½ cup coconut flour

1 cup arrowroot flour

1 teaspoon baking soda

⅓ cup unsweetened cocoa powder

2 tablespoons The Myers Way
    Gelatin (or similar gelatin)

2 teaspoons pure vanilla extract

1 avocado, pitted and chopped
    into pieces

½ cup maple syrup

1¼ cups filtered water

¼ cup palm shortening

Grease an 8-by-8-inch glass baking dish with either coconut oil or palm shortening.

Heat oven to 350°F. In the bowl of an electric mixer, combine the coconut and arrowroot flours, baking soda, cocoa powder, and gelatin. On low speed, mix the dry ingredients together. Add the remaining ingredients. Beat with mixer until batter is formed.

Pour batter into the prepared dish and spread evenly. Bake for 35 to 40 minutes or until a toothpick comes out clean. Remove from oven and let cool for 5 minutes before cutting into bars.

Lemon Bars

Makes 9 bars

It's a tough call when choosing between a Fudgy Brownie (page 232) and these lemon bars. They have just enough sweetness to balance the tart lemony flavor.

Crust
- 1 cup coconut flour
- ¼ cup arrowroot flour
- 1⅓ cups palm shortening
- ¼ cup maple syrup

Filling
- 1⅓ cups freshly squeezed lemon juice
- 1 cup coconut sugar
- Pinch of ground turmeric
- 1½ cups coconut cream
- ¼ cup arrowroot flour

Heat oven to 350°F. Grease an 8-by-8-inch baking dish with coconut oil.

In the bowl of an electric mixer, mix together the coconut flour and arrowroot flour. Add the palm shortening and maple syrup and beat on low until the dough comes together. Using your fingers, gently press the dough into the bottom of the prepared dish.

Bake for 10 minutes. Remove the pan from the oven and lower the temperature to 325°F.

In the bowl of an electric mixer, beat together lemon juice, coconut sugar, turmeric, coconut cream, and arrowroot flour on medium speed until combined. Pour on top of the crust. Bake for 20 minutes or until filling starts to set (filling will set more when it's refrigerated). Remove from oven and let the bars cool for 10 minutes. Refrigerate for 30 minutes and allow to set completely before serving. Slice into bars.

Birthday Cupcakes

Makes 18 cupcakes

We celebrated Elle's first birthday with a tower of these colorful cupcakes frosted with chocolate, maple-cinnamon, and strawberry icings. Most of the guests at our one-year-old's party were grown-ups, though you'd never know it, given the way they gobbled up these cupcakes!

Cupcakes

1⅓ cups cassava flour

½ cup coconut flour

¼ cup arrowroot flour

4 teaspoons baking soda

4 teaspoons cream of tartar

1½ cups coconut sugar

2 tablespoons The Myers Way Gelatin (or similar gelatin)

¾ cup palm shortening

2 tablespoons pure vanilla extract

½ cup unsweetened applesauce

2 teaspoons apple cider vinegar

1½ cups full-fat coconut milk

Icing

Makes 3 cups

3 cups palm shortening

⅓ cup coconut oil

2 tablespoons pure vanilla extract

¾ teaspoon powdered stevia

2 tablespoons maple syrup

1 tablespoon tapioca starch

Chocolate Icing:

Add 2 tablespoons cocoa powder and 1 tablespoon maple syrup when beating the icing.

Maple-Cinnamon Icing:

Add 2 tablespoons maple syrup and 1½ teaspoons ground cinnamon when beating the icing.

Strawberry Icing:

Add 1½ cups chopped fresh strawberries when beating the icing.

Heat oven to 350°F. Place a paper cupcake liner in each muffin pan cup or arrange 18 silicone muffin cups on a sheet pan.

To make the cupcakes: In the bowl of an electric mixer, mix together the cassava flour, coconut flour, arrowroot flour, baking soda, cream of tartar, coconut sugar, and gelatin on low speed. Add palm shortening, vanilla, applesauce, vinegar, and coconut milk. Beat on low, then medium speed, scraping down the sides, until well mixed.

Fill each muffin cup two-thirds full with batter. Lightly press dough down into the cup. Bake for 20 minutes or until a toothpick inserted in the center of one or two cupcakes comes out clean. Let the cupcakes cool completely before icing.

To make the icing: In the bowl of an electric mixer, beat the palm shortening and coconut oil on low until combined. Add vanilla, stevia, maple syrup, and tapioca starch. Beat on low for 1 minute, then increase the speed to medium-high and beat until smooth and thoroughly combined.

Dark Chocolate Bark

Makes 10 to 12 pieces

This thin, delicate treat can satisfy your chocolate cravings without sabotaging your waistline. The Myers Way Collagen Protein will give you a protein and energy boost. You can add any ingredients you want to this bark. When it's ready to eat, break off a piece to enjoy. Then another . . . and another . . .

1 cup coconut oil

1½ cups unsweetened cocoa
    powder

1 teaspoon stevia

2 scoops The Myers Way Collagen
    Protein (or similar collagen)

Optional Toppings: Freeze-dried
    fruit, toasted unsweetened
    coconut chips, coarse sea salt

Line a sheet pan with parchment paper.

Melt the coconut oil in a saucepan over low heat. Remove saucepan from heat and add the cocoa powder, stevia, and collagen. Stir to combine.

Pour the chocolate mixture onto the prepared pan. Sprinkle on toppings of your choice. Refrigerate for 30 minutes, until firm. Break into pieces to serve.

Raspberry Cheesecake Bites

Makes 12

If you're like me, you don't have time to spend hours making desserts, yet sometimes you need something sweet for a dinner or just for yourself. These cheesecakey bites are creamy and light. Add The Myers Way Collagen Protein for a protein and energy boost, as well as its gut-repairing properties.

Cheesecake

¾ cup coconut butter

¾ cup fresh raspberries

2 dates

⅛ teaspoon ground cinnamon

⅛ teaspoon ground ginger

1 teaspoon lemon zest

1 scoop The Myers Way Collagen
   Protein (optional)

Optional Icing

¼ cup coconut oil

2 scoops The Myers Way Vanilla
   Paleo Protein (or similar
   protein powder)

To make the cheesecake bites: Put all ingredients in the bowl of a food processor. Pulse until blended. Using clean hands, form 1-inch balls and arrange on a plate in a single layer. Refrigerate for 10 to 15 minutes.

To make the icing: In a saucepan over medium heat, melt the coconut oil. Remove from heat and whisk in the protein powder.

Remove cheesecake bites from refrigerator. Dip them in the icing or drizzle the icing over the tops. Return bites to the refrigerator and allow the icing to solidify for 10 to 15 minutes.

Chocolate Whoopie Pies

Makes 4 3-inch whoopie pies

Creamy icing is sandwiched between two dark chocolate cakes in this American classic. Whoopie pies are half cake and half cookie and all delicious. Use the Chocolate Icing from the Birthday Cupcakes (page 234), although you may not need all of it.

⅔ cup cassava flour

¼ cup coconut flour

2 tablespoons arrowroot flour

½ cup unsweetened cocoa powder

½ cup coconut sugar

2 teaspoons baking soda

2 teaspoons cream of tartar

1 tablespoon The Myers Way Gelatin (or similar gelatin)

1 cup full-fat coconut milk

½ cup unsweetened applesauce

2 tablespoons pure vanilla extract

2 teaspoons apple cider vinegar

½ cup palm shortening

Chocolate Icing (page 234)

Heat oven to 350°F. Line two sheet pans with parchment paper.

In the bowl of an electric mixer, mix together the cassava flour, coconut flour, arrowroot flour, cocoa, sugar, baking soda, cream of tartar, and gelatin on low speed.

In a separate bowl, whisk together the coconut milk, applesauce, vanilla, and vinegar. Add the liquid ingredients to the mixing bowl and beat on low, then medium speed, scraping down the sides, until well mixed. Add in the shortening and combine.

Using clean hands, form the dough into eight 1-inch balls and place on prepared pans. Flatten the dough balls with the palm of your hand into 3-inch rounds. Bake for 10 minutes, or until a toothpick inserted into the middle of a cookie comes out clean. Remove cookies from oven and let cool.

While the cookies are baking, prepare the icing. Spread 1 to 2 tablespoons icing onto four of the cookies and then top each with another cookie.

Creamy Frozen Fruit Pops

Makes 6 popsicles

Kids will never know these popsicles are so healthy. They are so sweet and creamy that kids will be begging for another. These popsicles make for a wonderful after-dinner or poolside treat. For more traditional and less creamy popsicles, you can swap out the coconut milk for coconut water or filtered water.

2 cups frozen strawberries

2 cups frozen mango

1 can full-fat coconut milk, divided

Place strawberries and ½ can coconut milk in a blender and blend until smooth. Remove from blender and add mangos and remaining coconut milk and blend until smooth.

In popsicle molds or small paper cups, alternate strawberry and mango layers. Insert popsicle base or a stick in each and place in freezer. Chill for 1 hour or until hardened.

Run popsicle molds or cups under warm water to loosen.

Pumpkin Pie

Serves 8

When someone asks you whether you can bring a pumpkin pie to a holiday dinner, now you can say, "Of course!" The crust is made with coconut and arrowroot flours and the filling with canned organic pumpkin puree, which is available year-round. A reminder: buy pumpkin puree rather than pumpkin pie filling, which has added sugars. When cooled, top this pie with Vanilla Cinnamon Coconut Mousse (page 245).

Crust

- 1 cup plus 2 tablespoons coconut flour
- 3 tablespoons arrowroot flour, plus extra for dusting
- ¾ cup coconut oil
- 3 tablespoons maple syrup

Filling

- 1 15-ounce can organic pumpkin puree
- 1½ cups full-fat coconut milk
- ¾ cup coconut sugar
- 2 teaspoons arrowroot flour
- 2 teaspoons pure vanilla extract
- ¾ teaspoon ground cinnamon
- ½ teaspoon ground nutmeg
- ½ teaspoon ground ginger
- ¼ teaspoon ground cloves
- 1 teaspoon fine sea salt

To make the crust: Heat oven to 350°F. In a mixer, combine crust ingredients on low until a dough is formed. Shape the dough into a ball, wrap in plastic wrap, and place in refrigerator for 10 minutes.

While dough is chilling, combine filling ingredients in the bowl of a mixer with whisk attachment. Beat until all ingredients are combined.

Remove the dough from the refrigerator. Dust a work surface with a little arrowroot flour. Roll out the dough to fit a 9-inch glass pie plate. If the dough cracks, reform with fingers. Transfer crust to a greased pie dish and remove any extra crust.

Bake the crust for 5 minutes, or until lightly browned. Remove from the oven and increase oven temperature to 375°F. Evenly pour in the filling. Bake for 45 to 50 minutes, or until filling has solidified. Remove the pie from oven and let cool on a wire rack. Place in the refrigerator and serve cold.

Banana Pudding

Serves 12

This banana pudding is as easy as pie and is a Myers family favorite. A rich banana filling is layered with a sweet, crunchy, and crumbly topping.

Filling

- 3 cups full-fat coconut milk, divided
- 1 tablespoon pure vanilla extract
- 2 teaspoons The Myers Way Gelatin (or similar gelatin)
- 4 ripe bananas
- 1 tablespoon maple syrup

Crumble

- ¼ cup tigernut flour
- ½ cup coconut flour
- ⅛ teaspoon fine sea salt
- ¼ teaspoon baking soda
- 1 teaspoon ground cinnamon
- ¼ cup coconut oil, melted
- ¼ cup honey
- 1 teaspoon pure vanilla extract

To make the filling: In a saucepan, bring 2 cups coconut milk and vanilla to a simmer. In a separate bowl, whisk together the remaining 1 cup coconut milk with the gelatin. Remove saucepan from the heat and whisk in gelatin mixture. Transfer to a glass storage container and refrigerate the pudding until set, about 3 hours.

While the pudding sets, heat oven to 350°F. Line a sheet pan with parchment paper.

To make the crumble: In a bowl, combine the tigernut and coconut flours, salt, baking soda, cinnamon, coconut oil, honey, and vanilla until it holds together. Press the dough into the prepared pan to a ¼-inch thickness. Bake for 15 minutes until lightly browned. Let cool, then crumble into small bites.

In the bowl of an electric mixer on medium speed, beat together two bananas and maple syrup until mashed. Add half the pudding and mix well. Add the remaining pudding and mix until fully combined.

Evenly scatter a third of the crumble on the bottom of an 8-by-8-inch baking dish. Slice one banana and arrange it on top of the crumble. Pour on half of the pudding mixture. Repeat with the crumble, one banana, and pudding. Top with the remaining crumble. Refrigerate for 30 minutes before serving.

Apple Crisp

Serves 6

Thanks to tigernuts, the sky's the limit when it comes to making desserts. Whole tigernuts and tigernut flour are used in this fruit classic. Tigernuts are loaded with prebiotics, which are low in sugar and important for great gut health. No apples? Substitute an equal amount of pears or 2 to 3 cups of mixed fresh or frozen berries.

Fruit Filling

4 medium apples, chopped

2 tablespoons tigernut flour

Juice of ½ lemon

½ teaspoon ground cinnamon

¼ teaspoon ground nutmeg

Topping

1½ cups slivered tigernuts

¾ cup coconut sugar

¼ cup tigernut flour

4 tablespoons palm shortening

1 teaspoon pure vanilla extract

½ teaspoon ground cinnamon

⅛ teaspoon fine sea salt

Heat oven to 375°F.

To make the filling: In a bowl, mix together apples, flour, lemon juice, cinnamon, and nutmeg. Pour into an 8-by-8-inch baking dish.

To make the topping: In a separate bowl, use a fork to mix the tigernuts, sugar, tigernut flour, shortening, vanilla, cinnamon, and salt into a crumbly topping. Evenly sprinkle the topping over the apples. Bake for 35 to 40 minutes, or until topping is lightly browned. Serve warm.

Coconut Chocolate Mousse

Serves 4

I have received so many emails from readers of The Autoimmune Solution *raving about this dessert that I just had to include an adapted version of it here. Traditional chocolate mousse requires separating eggs and melting chocolate. My dairy-free mousse requires just one bowl for mixing, so it's ready in no time.*

2 13.5-ounce cans full-fat coconut milk, refrigerated overnight

2 tablespoons unsweetened cocoa powder

1 teaspoon pure vanilla extract

10 to 15 drops liquid stevia

½ teaspoon ground cinnamon

¼ teaspoon fine sea salt

Fresh berries (optional)

Unsweetened coconut flakes (optional)

Skim off the top layer of the coconut cream and place in a bowl, leaving behind the watery "milk" in the can for another use.

Using a hand whisk or electric mixer, beat the coconut cream into a mousse-like consistency. If you would like, reserve some cream before adding cocoa, to top the mousse before serving.

With a spoon, mix in cocoa, vanilla, stevia, cinnamon, and salt. Put in a serving bowl. Garnish with berries, coconut flakes, or reserved coconut cream.

Vanilla Cinnamon: Omit the cocoa powder and increase cinnamon to 1 teaspoon.

"Peanut Butter" Cups

Makes 12

Reese's peanut butter cups were my favorite candy when I was growing up. My parents were very health conscious so I was allowed to eat them only at Easter and Halloween. With this healthier version, you don't have to limit yourself to enjoying them only twice a year. They're rich, chocolaty, nutty, and irresistible. And they are so easy to make in one pan.

½ cup coconut oil

1 cup unsweetened cocoa powder

½ teaspoon stevia

2 scoops The Myers Way Collagen
    Protein (or similar protein)

¼ cup Tigernut Butter (page 219) or
    Coconut Butter (page 69)

Melt the coconut oil in a saucepan. Whisk in the cocoa powder, stevia, and collagen until combined.

Pour a spoonful of chocolate mixture into each cup of a paper-lined regular-size muffin tin. Add 1 teaspoon of Tigernut Butter or Coconut Butter. Cover with the remaining chocolate.

Refrigerate until solid, about 30 minutes.

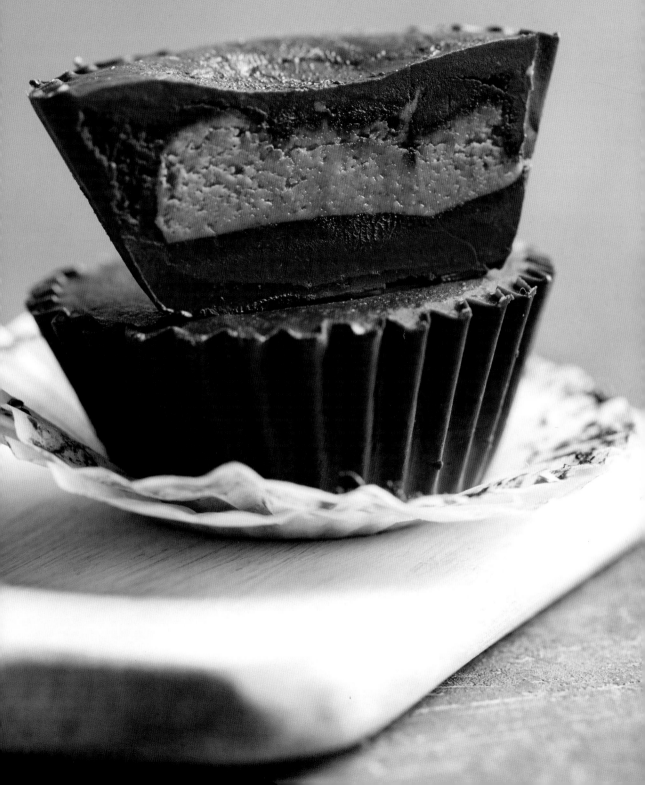

"Peanut Butter" Cups, page 246

Gingerbread Cake, page 230

Lemon Bars,
page 233

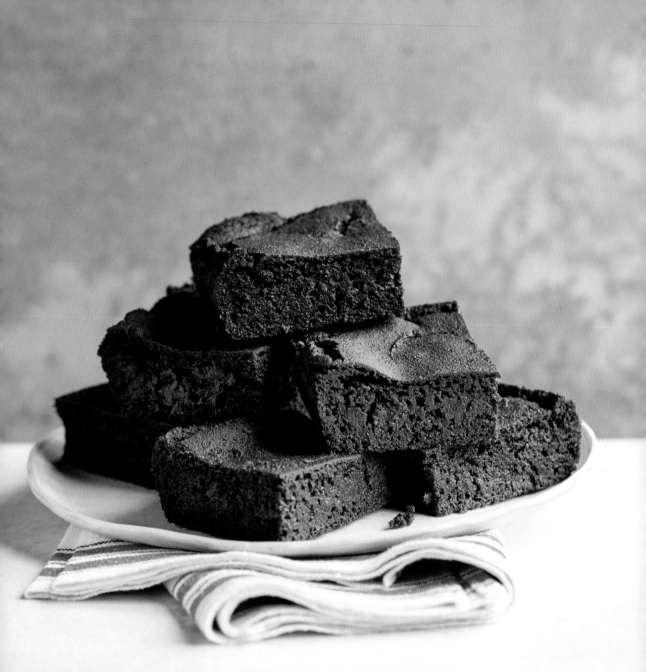

Fudgy Brownies, page 232

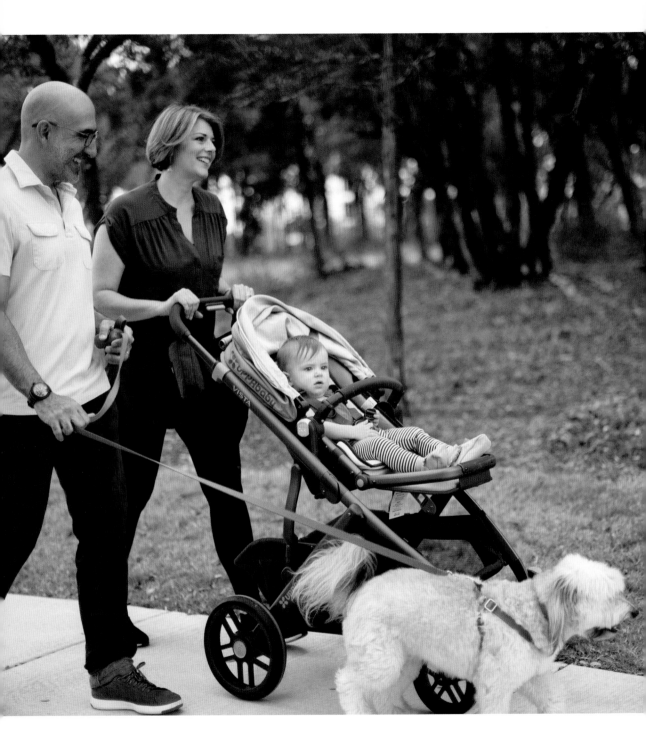

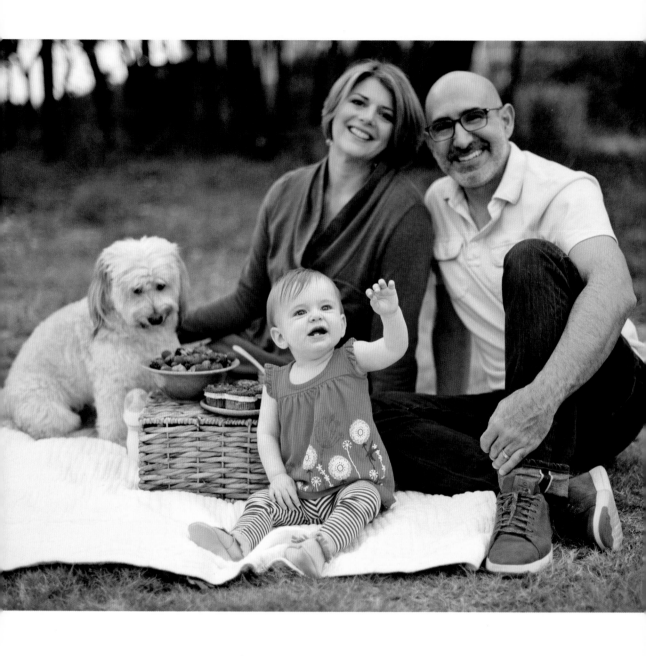

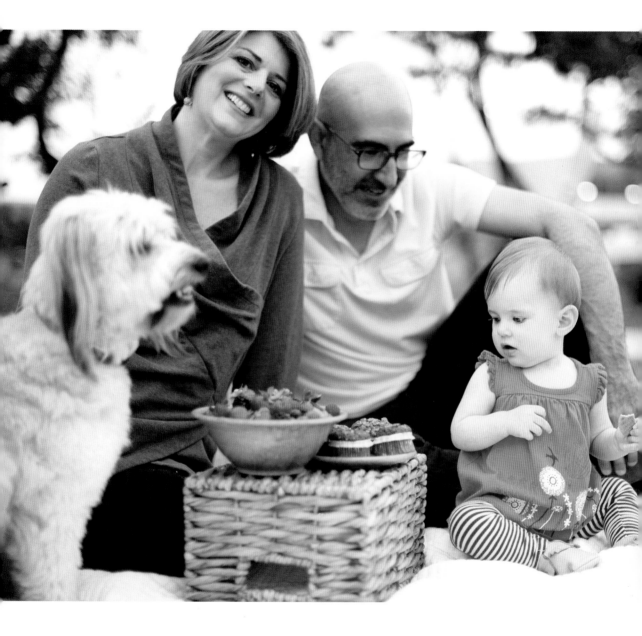

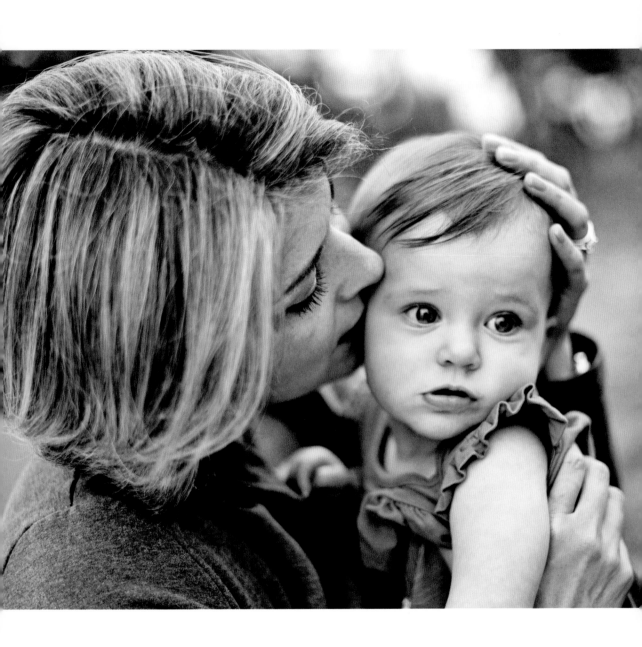

Specific Diet Chart

✓ = Approved for specific diet

	Autoimmune Friendly	Thyroid Friendly	Candida	SIBO*	Low Histamine†
STAPLE RECIPES					
Caramelized Onions	✓	✓	✓		
Cauliflower Rice	✓	✓	✓	✓	
Coconut Butter	✓	✓	✓	✓	
Coconut Milk	✓	✓	✓	✓	
Coconut Milk Yogurt	✓	✓	✓	✓	
Gut-Healing Bone Broth	✓	✓	✓		
Roasted Garlic	✓	✓	✓		
BREAKFAST					
Acai Smoothie Bowl	✓	✓			
BLC Tacos	✓	✓	✓	✓	
Cassava Tortillas	✓	✓			✓
Coconut Yogurt Parfaits	✓	✓			
Crunchy Maple Granola	✓	✓			
Pumpkin Pancakes	✓	✓			✓
Roasted Sweet Potato Rounds with Smoked Salmon	✓	✓	✓	✓	

*If you have SIBO and are sensitive to garlic and/or onion, simply remove any from a recipe to make that recipe SIBO friendly.
†See "Note on Histamine Intolerance" on page 255.

	Autoimmune Friendly	Thyroid Friendly	Candida	SIBO*	Low Histamine†
Savory Breakfast Sausage	✓	✓	✓	✓	✓
Spaghetti Squash Hash Browns	✓	✓	✓	✓	✓
Sweet Potato–Bacon Hash with Avocado Cream	✓	✓	✓	✓	
Sweet Potato Biscuits	✓	✓			✓
Tigernut Oatmeal	✓	✓			
Tigernut Waffles	✓	✓			✓
Turkey-Butternut Squash Hash	✓	✓	✓	✓	✓
Zucchini Muffins	✓	✓			

SMOOTHIES, JUICES, AND OTHER BEVERAGES

	Autoimmune Friendly	Thyroid Friendly	Candida	SIBO*	Low Histamine†
Agua Fresca	✓	✓			
Blackberry-Basil Mule	✓	✓			
Chai Smoothie	✓	✓	✓	✓	
Chai Tea Latte	✓	✓			✓
Cherry Sunrise Smoothie	✓	✓			✓
Classic Detoxifying Green Juice	✓				
Creamy Hot Chocolate	✓	✓	✓	✓	
Dark Chocolate–Cherry Smoothie	✓	✓	✓	✓	
Free-Radical Fighter	✓	✓			
French Vanilla Coffee Creamer	✓	✓	✓	✓	✓
Gingerbread Cookie Smoothie	✓	✓			

	Autoimmune Friendly	Thyroid Friendly	Candida	SIBO*	Low Histamine†
Golden Milk	✓	✓	✓	✓	✓
Gut-Soothing Collagen Tea	✓	✓	✓	✓	
Kale–Mint–Lemongrass Smoothie	✓		✓	✓	
Mean Green Smoothie	✓	✓	✓	✓	
Mint–Chocolate Chip Smoothie	✓	✓	✓	✓	
Organic Green Margarita Juice	✓	✓			
Peppermint Hot Chocolate	✓	✓	✓	✓	
Pumpkin Pie Smoothie	✓	✓	✓	✓	
Pumpkin Spice Latte	✓	✓			✓
Purple Perfection	✓	✓			
Rosemary-Lemon Spritzer	✓	✓	✓	✓	
Sangria	✓	✓			
Splash of Sunshine	✓	✓			
Strawberry Cheesecake Smoothie	✓	✓	✓	✓	
Strawberry Mojito	✓	✓	✓	✓	
Tropical Green Smoothie	✓	✓			
Very Berry Smoothie	✓	✓	✓	✓	✓
SOUPS AND SALADS					
Apricot-Chicken Salad	✓	✓			
Brussels Sprouts and Red Cabbage Salad	✓				

	Autoimmune Friendly	Thyroid Friendly	Candida	SIBO*	Low Histamine†
Butternut Squash–Sage Soup	✓	✓	✓	✓	
Cauliflower Chowder	✓	✓	✓	✓	
Chicken "Noodle" Soup	✓	✓	✓	✓	
Chicken Tortilla Soup	✓	✓	✓	✓	
Creamy Zucchini-Basil Soup	✓	✓	✓	✓	
Cucumber-Seaweed Salad	✓	✓			
Curried Carrot Soup	✓	✓	✓	✓	
Herbed "Potato" Salad	✓	✓	✓	✓	
Mardi Gras Salad	✓	✓	✓	✓	✓
Roasted Vegetable Soup	✓	✓	✓	✓	
Tangy Coleslaw	✓				
Thai Meatball Soup	✓	✓			
Tropical Nicaraguan Salad	✓	✓			
Winter Salad with Maple Vinaigrette	✓			✓	
MAIN COURSES					
Apple-Stuffed Pork Chops with Maple Glaze	✓	✓		✓	
Baked Chicken and Sweet Potatoes with Lemon-Rosemary Sauce	✓	✓	✓	✓	
Bison Chili	✓	✓	✓	✓	
Braised Pork Ribs	✓	✓		✓	

	Autoimmune Friendly	Thyroid Friendly	Candida	SIBO*	Low Histamine†
Carolina Pulled Pork	✓	✓	✓	✓	
Chicken Burrito Bowl	✓	✓	✓	✓	✓
Chicken Nuggets	✓	✓	✓	✓	✓
Chicken Pad Thai	✓	✓			
Chicken Rollatini with Bacon and Pesto	✓	✓	✓	✓	
Chimichurri Lamb Kebobs	✓	✓	✓	✓	
Coconut Shrimp	✓	✓			
Create Your Own Coconut Curry	✓	✓	✓	✓	✓
Halibut Piccata	✓	✓	✓	✓	
Herb Roasted Chicken	✓	✓	✓	✓	✓
Honey-Ginger Glazed Salmon	✓	✓		✓	
Lamb Chops with Cherry Glaze	✓	✓			
Lamb Meatballs in Lettuce Wraps	✓	✓	✓	✓	
Meatballs	✓	✓	✓	✓	✓
Mississippi Roast	✓	✓	✓	✓	
Mushroom and Asparagus Caulisotto	✓	✓			
Perfect Fast Man Burgers	✓	✓	✓	✓	✓
Pesto Pizza	✓	✓			
Pork Tenderloin with Mustard Sauce	✓	✓	✓	✓	
Turkey Pot Pie	✓	✓	✓	✓	

	Autoimmune Friendly	Thyroid Friendly	Candida	SIBO*	Low Histamine†
Vegetable Fried "Rice"	✓	✓			
World's Best Asian Flank Steak	✓	✓			
SIDES					
Bacon-Wrapped Asparagus	✓	✓	✓	✓	
Broccolini with Garlic and Lemon	✓	✓	✓*	✓	
Cauliflower Saffron "Rice"	✓	✓	✓	✓	
Creamy Vegetables "Alfredo"	✓	✓	✓	✓	✓
Grilled Bok Choy	✓	✓			
Loaded and Baked Sweet Potatoes	✓	✓	✓	✓	✓
Mashed Cauliflower and Rutabaga	✓	✓	✓	✓	✓
Roasted Brussels Sprouts with Bacon	✓	✓			✓
Roasted Vegetables	✓	✓	✓	✓	✓
Root Vegetable Pancakes	✓	✓	✓	✓	✓
Sweet Potato Fries	✓	✓	✓	✓	✓
Wilted Greens with Bacon	✓	✓	✓	✓	
Zucchini Noodles with Spinach-Kale Pesto	✓	✓	✓	✓	
DRESSINGS, SAUCES, AND CONDIMENTS					
Aïoli	✓	✓	✓	✓	
Apple-Cinnamon Compote	✓	✓			
Betty's Italian Dressing	✓	✓		✓	

	Autoimmune Friendly	Thyroid Friendly	Candida	SIBO*	Low Histamine†
Blackberry Vinaigrette	✓	✓			
Blueberry-Lemon Compote	✓	✓			
Caramelized Banana Compote	✓	✓			
Cherry Barbecue Sauce	✓	✓			
Green Goddess Dressing	✓	✓	✓	✓	
Herbed Vinaigrette	✓	✓	✓	✓	
Ketchup	✓	✓	✓	✓	
Mango-Avocado Salsa	✓	✓			
Meat Marinade	✓	✓			
No-Mato Sauce	✓	✓	✓	✓	
"Peanut" Sauce	✓	✓			
Ranch Dressing	✓	✓			
Spinach-Kale Pesto	✓	✓		✓	
Tapenade	✓	✓	✓	✓	
Tzatziki	✓	✓	✓	✓	
World's Best Asian Marinade	✓	✓			
SNACKS					
Beef Jerky	✓	✓	✓	✓	
Chicken Satay with "Peanut" Sauce	✓	✓			
Coconut Collagen Fuel Bites	✓	✓	✓	✓	✓

	Autoimmune Friendly	Thyroid Friendly	Candida	SIBO*	Low Histamine†
Five-Vegetable Guacamole	✓	✓	✓	✓	✓
Fruit Snacks	✓	✓	✓	✓	
Plantain Chips	✓	✓	✓	✓	✓
Root Vegetable Chips	✓	✓	✓	✓	✓
Rosemary–Sea Salt Crackers	✓	✓			✓
Rutabaga "Hummus"	✓	✓	✓	✓	✓
Spinach-Artichoke Dip	✓	✓	✓	✓	
Sweet-and-Salty Trail Mix	✓	✓			
Tigernut Butter	✓	✓			✓
Wild-Caught Shrimp Sushi Rolls	✓	✓	✓	✓	
DESSERTS					
Anne's Amazing Cinnamon Raisin Cookies	✓	✓			✓
Apple Crisp	✓	✓			
Banana Pudding	✓	✓			
Birthday Cupcakes	✓	✓			✓
Chocolate Whoopie Pies	✓	✓			
Coconut Chocolate Mousse	✓	✓	✓	✓	✓
Creamy Frozen Fruit Pops	✓	✓	✓	✓	
Dark Chocolate Bark	✓	✓	✓	✓	
Fudgy Brownies	✓	✓			

	Autoimmune Friendly	Thyroid Friendly	Candida	SIBO*	Low Histamine†
Gingerbread Cake	✓	✓			
Lemon Bars	✓	✓			
"Peanut Butter" Cups	✓	✓	✓	✓	
Pumpkin Pie	✓	✓			
Raspberry Cheesecake Bites	✓	✓			

NOTE ON HISTAMINE INTOLERANCE

Histamine intolerance varies from person to person as histamines vary in amount from food to food. Certain foods are naturally high in histamines; here are the big culprits:

Apple cider vinegar	Coconut aminos
Avocado	Dried fruits
Bacon	Fish sauce
Bananas	Olives
Bone broth	Shellfish
Citrus	Spinach
Cocoa	Strawberries

Some of the recipes approved for "Low Histamine" diets may contain some of these foods; however, these recipes can easily be made without the high-histamine ingredients. Simply remove them from the recipe altogether to make "Low Histamine"!

SIBO can often be a root cause of histamine intolerance. To determine whether you have SIBO, visit amymd.io/quiz.

12

___

Home and Body

Did you know that your beauty products and household cleaners likely contain toxic chemicals that disrupt your immune system?

More than eighty thousand chemicals are in use in the United States, and the vast majority haven't been tested for safety. On top of that, most products contain a number of toxic chemicals that haven't even been tested for safety in isolation, much less in combination with others.

The beauty industry has a particularly ugly side because all cosmetic ingredients are reviewed for safety by the Cosmetic Ingredient Review (CIR), an industry-appointed and industry-funded panel, rather than by an independent agency such as the Food and Drug Administration (FDA).

Since Tame the Toxins is the third pillar of The Myers Way, I'm including this chapter on how to make your own toxin-free body and cleaning products. They are simple to make and cost far less than the store-bought versions, so you'll be protecting your and your family's health and saving money at the same time!

For products that I can't make, I order toxin-free makeup and bath and beauty products from Beautycounter (see Resources).

It's important to make sure you switch to nontoxic products as part of The Myers Way because toxins play such a huge role in your immune system and overall health.

Stress-Relieving Lavender Spa Bath Salts

Makes 1¼ cups

Relieve Your Stress is part of the fourth pillar of The Myers Way, and with these spa bath salts, that is easy to do! They are simple to make and they won't break the bank like most commercial spa bath salts. I take a hot bath with these salts almost every night. Feel free to experiment and try other essential oils that relieve stress for you.

1 cup Epsom salts

¼ cup baking soda

1 tablespoon coarse sea salt

10 drops organic lavender oil

Combine all ingredients in a glass container with a tight-fitting lid. Shake well. Add ¼ cup to your bath water.

Lemongrass Natural Deodorant

Makes ½ cup

This fabulous-smelling deodorant works great in the hot Texas summers—so it should work anywhere! By making this natural deodorant, you skip the toxins and save money.

¼ cup baking soda

¼ cup arrowroot starch

6 tablespoons coconut oil

Lemongrass essential oil or any essential oil of your choosing (optional)

Mix baking soda and arrowroot starch together in a bowl. Add coconut oil and mash the ingredients together with a fork. Add a few drops of essential oils, if desired. Store in a small glass jar for easy use. To use, swipe two fingers into the deodorant and apply to armpits.

Toothpaste

You won't believe how smooth and clean your teeth feel after using this all-natural and toxin-free toothpaste. You can make this as a powder or a paste.

½ cup baking soda

1 teaspoon fine sea salt

Hydrogen peroxide, 3 percent

Filtered water

1 tablespoon coconut oil (optional)

2 to 6 drops peppermint essential
   oil (optional)

In a glass jar, mix baking soda and sea salt. In a separate dark glass bottle, mix 1 part hydrogen peroxide and 1 part filtered water. Dip your toothbrush in the hydrogen peroxide–water mixture, then dip it into the baking soda mixture and brush your teeth.

To make a paste, mix coconut oil and essential oil into the baking soda and sea salt.

All-Purpose Cleaner

Make 2¼ cups

We use only homemade cleaners in our house. They are free of toxins and clean even the toughest of messes.

2 cups filtered water

¼ cup liquid Castile soap

10 drops essential oil, such as lemon, tea tree, or peppermint

Mix all ingredients together in a glass spray bottle. Shake well before using.

Bath and Sink Scrub

Makes 3 cups

This easy cleaning scrub works just as well as anything you can buy in the store—and it's toxin-free!

1 cup baking soda

10 drops essential oil, such as
   lemon, tea tree, or peppermint

¼ cup liquid Castile soap

2 cups filtered water

In a glass container, mix baking soda and essential oil. Mix the Castile soap and water in a 24-ounce spray bottle. When ready to use, shake the bottle well. Sprinkle the baking soda mixture on the surface to be cleaned, then spray the soap mixture on the surface and scrub with a bristle brush or sponge.

Glass Cleaner

Makes 2¼ cups

Use this cleaner for tabletops, mirrors, and windows. It will leave them bright and clear.

2 cups filtered water

2 tablespoons white vinegar

2 tablespoons rubbing alcohol

5 drops peppermint essential oil

Mix all ingredients together in a 24-ounce spray bottle. Shake well before using.

Part Four

The Myers Way® for Life

13

Getting the Whole Family on Board

I was raised eating real whole foods. We shopped at the local natural foods store (this was before there was a Whole Foods Market), had a garden, grew sprouts, and made our own yogurt. My mom taught me how to bake, and my dad taught me how to cook. I learned how to be involved with the food that I put in my body and understood that it was meant to nourish me. I dedicated this book to my parents because they instilled in me the importance of a nourishing diet and real whole foods. Although it turned out that the type of food I was eating (a vegetarian diet of grains, legumes, and dairy) wasn't good for me because of my predisposition toward autoimmunity, I will always be grateful to my parents for teaching me how to be involved with my food in a way that many of my peers were not and many children these days are not.

What I wish for you (and for your families and your friends!) is for you to see food as a tool for healing and to commit to making informed choices when it comes to the food that you eat so that you can get your health back and stay well. My suggestions for how to bring The Myers Way into your life are a little different from those you might pick up from another cookbook or "diet" book. I'm not going to suggest that you "ease off" sometimes or have "cheat" days or "treat yourself" to a gooey, gluten-filled cupcake on your birthday. *The Myers Way is not a diet. It is a way of life.* This is a vital distinction, because autoimmunity impacts our short-term and long-term well-being. This is not a weight-loss program where a cheat day is okay because the consequence is an extra lingering pound or two. Once we identify the symptoms of autoimmunity, finding the root cause and living the solution is vital for moving to the healthy end of the autoimmune spectrum and staying there.

Most of you reading this book are likely women, and many of you are moms, since women are three times more likely than men to develop autoimmune conditions, and those conditions often develop during or after pregnancy. As women and mothers, you are likely used to putting everyone and everything else first—your children, your partner, your parents. I'm a mom, wife, physician, and business owner, so I get it! However, and I want you to really internalize this: this is the moment when you need to *put yourself first*. Remember, the very best way for you to be there for your family is if you are healthy, happy, and whole. By committing to *your* health, you are truly supporting everyone. And the easiest way to maintain that commitment is to get your whole family on board.

Getting Your Family to Appreciate Nourishing Foods

Explain to your family that you will be changing the way you eat by enjoying delicious, real foods with the power to nourish everyone's bodies and improve everyone's health. Rather than thinking of this as asking your family to give up certain foods, think about it in terms of the health benefits they'll be gaining. While your family members may initially get on board simply out of solidarity, once they see the positive changes from following The Myers Way, you will see them sticking with the program for their own personal health. Women often tell me that their partners lose weight, think more clearly, and have more energy and that their children are more focused in school, have fewer emotional outbursts, and their behavioral issues vanish—all by switching to The Myers Way.

Not to mention that you want the very best for your children, and making eating for optimal health a way of life when they are young is much easier than trying to make the switch when they are in their teens or twenties. Again, this is something I will always be grateful for with my own parents because it meant that once I finally figured out what diet worked best for reversing autoimmunity, I wasn't switching abruptly from packaged junk foods to broccoli; I was still eating broccoli and simply swapping out whole grains for lean, organic grass-fed meats.

And now I have the joy of instilling that same appreciation for nourishing foods in my own daughter. I cook only The Myers Way meals for my family, and Xavier and Elle, who do not have autoimmune issues, love every bite. Rather than rice cereal, Elle's first solid food was an organic avocado, and she has never had gluten or cow's milk. Elle was breastfed for the first ten months and now drinks camel's milk and eats grass-fed, pasture-raised meats and organic vegetables and fruits. She doesn't have an autoimmune disorder, and by eating this way, I am hoping she never will. Elle is thriving, and we eat together as a family every night, enjoying many of the recipes in this book.

Remember, The Myers Way isn't about deprivation—you will be enjoying delicious, flavorful foods that will keep you energized and full. It may take a few days to fully adjust to the changes, but just remember: you, your partner, and your children were designed to thrive on real, whole foods, and you're making a powerful investment in their health as well as yours.

Beginning Step by Step

If you or a family member does not have autoimmunity and you just want to improve your diet to prevent health issues, you can go slowly if you, your partner, or your child is a particularly picky eater. (I went through a phase when I was about twelve years old where I would eat only white rice and cottage cheese—so trust me, I get it!) For example, if your child's go-to food is macaroni and cheese out of a box, start by switching to a gluten-free, dairy-free version. Another great introduction is for everyone to start the day with a delicious smoothie, featuring The Myers Way Paleo Protein to keep them full and energized until lunch. Your child can even pick out his or her own ingredients to be involved in the process.

If your child (or even your partner!) is used to packing a sandwich for lunch, you can first switch to gluten-free bread and then move on to using more autoimmune-friendly Cassava Tortillas (page 100) or lettuce for wraps.

And this same principle applies to desserts and sweet treats. Swap your dairy-filled ice cream for a dairy-free alternative, and then move to Creamy Frozen Fruit Pops (page 239) or Coconut Chocolate Mousse (page 245) blended to ice cream consistency for a frozen treat.

As you make these shifts, keep your house stocked with healthy snacks and wholesome foods—cooked chicken, roasted sweet potatoes and toppings, bowls of berries, Coconut Milk Yogurt (page 70). If your family members are hungry, they will eat it.

Pick Your Battles

Too many restrictions—whether associated with homework, bedtime, or food—can make kids feel like outsiders or want to rebel against any limitations whatsoever. Fighting peer pressure ("Emma's family eats pasta with tomato sauce . . ."), advertising, ("Kids, try this new cereal . . ."), and even just busy schedules will always take some effort. The key is to pick your battles. Are you okay with your family members ordering what they want in a restaurant, yet bringing only healthy foods into your home? Or are you okay if your child eats the "regular" cupcake at a birthday party? Only you and your family can decide what guidelines work best.

For example, I buy all organic food for cooking at home, and I do my best to find restaurants that use organic ingredients; however, sometimes that's simply not an option, so I eat produce or meats that aren't organic. I also drink only filtered water at home and in my office, and I take my glass bottle with me wherever I go; however, when I'm in a foreign country in a rural area and the only safe water to drink is in a plastic bottle, I drink that water. We don't live in a perfect world, and there will be times where you make concessions; it's all about making informed choices and finding a balance. I know my "absolute no" foods, which I never eat, and make compromises when I need to.

14

Travel Tips

Since I travel frequently, it's just as important that I maintain my healthy lifestyle on the road as I do at home. My number one travel recommendation is this: *Always be prepared*.

Pack Snacks and Meals. There's no need to resort to unhealthy grab-and-go snacks or highly processed fast "food" when you can plan ahead and take your own snacks and meals. I always prepare a meal to take on a flight no matter how long or short it is because you never know whether there will be delays. Usually the person next to me on the flight looks longingly at my grilled, pasture-raised herb roasted chicken and brussels sprouts and bacon while they eat whatever they picked up in the airport or one of the snacks that pass for food on the airplane. My go-to snacks and meals include a green salad with leftover Herb Roasted Chicken (page 152), a small container of Rutabaga "Hummus" (page 217) with some Rosemary–Sea Salt Crackers (page 222), Beef Jerky (page 224), and some Sweet-and-Salty Trail Mix (page 214).

Most hotel rooms have small refrigerators where you can store your meals, snacks, and smoothie ingredients, and if there is a mini bar instead, you can remove the contents and use it as your personal refrigerator. Consider staying at an Airbnb home (Airbnb.com) for use of a full kitchen.

Stay Hydrated. Xavier and I take glass or stainless-steel water bottles everywhere we go, and Elle has a glass sippy cup that she uses when we travel. When flying, be sure to empty your water bottle before going through security, and then look for water filtration stations on the other side of security so that you can refill your water bottle with filtered water before boarding.

Take Protein. For easy, filling meals while traveling, I take along The Myers Way Paleo Protein powder so that I can whip up a nourishing, protein-packed smoothie on the go. I also take The Myers Way Collagen Protein, which can be added to virtually any drink, hot or cold, to provide a protein boost.

Carry Your Supplements with You. I recommend carrying all supplements and essential medications such as thyroid hormone (if you take it) in your carryon bag in case of delays or lost luggage so that you're never in a bind. I recommend four essential supplements (page 289) for everyone in the family to take so that you can maintain a strong foundation for optimal health wherever you are.

Pack Clean Bath and Beauty Products. Don't resort to using the toxin-filled bath products at hotels. I always take my own. I fill travel-size bottles with nontoxic soap, lotion, and shampoo. I make my own Lemongrass Natural Deodorant (page 259) and take nontoxic makeup. Beautycounter.com has an extensive line of makeup, shampoos, and lotions as well as one of the safest sunscreens on the market.

15

Dining Out

During the first thirty days of following *The Autoimmune Solution* program, I recommend that you cook all of your meals at home so you have complete control over what does and what doesn't go into your food. Though more and more restaurants are including organic ingredients in their dishes and offering farm-to-table, grass-fed, and pasture-raised meats, it is difficult to know 100 percent the ingredients in your meal unless you cook it yourself. If you know of a restaurant that is familiar with The Myers Way or an autoimmune paleo diet, and it can accommodate your requests, then go for it. But for most of you, cooking at home for the first thirty days of *The Autoimmune Solution* program will be your best choice.

If you have completed *The Autoimmune Solution* thirty-day protocol and you have reintroduced foods and are aware of what your "absolute no" foods are (see chapter 17), then you can begin to branch out and eat and enjoy foods in restaurants and at friends' homes. Here are a few of my favorite tips and tricks for eating out.

> **Before choosing a restaurant, check out the menu online.** If there's truly nothing you can eat on a menu—they serve only pizza, for instance— it's okay to suggest going to another restaurant! However, that's pretty rare, since most restaurants are happy to work with you. I often call ahead and speak with the chef if we are trying a new restaurant.

There's no need to be embarrassed to ask the manager or the server about ingredients or food preparation. You are the customer, and they are there to serve you. Remember that a smile, "please," and "thank you" always help too. If the server can't tell you whether the fish is sprinkled with breadcrumbs or what kind of oil was used for cooking, politely ask to speak with the chef who prepares the food.

Make your own salad dressing. Squeeze a bit of lemon juice and drizzle a little olive oil on your greens. Request that tomatoes and peppers be omitted from your salad.

Side dishes. In place of a potato, grain, or nightshade side dish, ask for steamed broccoli, asparagus, carrots, or other vegetable.

Request that your food be prepared without sauces. Sauces often contain butter, flour, sugar, or soy sauce. Ask that fish, chicken, or beef be grilled or broiled with olive oil instead of butter. The same goes for marinades, which often contain soy sauce, tomato-based ingredients, and spices such as paprika and cayenne. Make sure the meat you order hasn't been marinated before cooking.

For sautéed foods, ask the kitchen to use olive oil instead of butter. Remind the server that you can eat only gluten-free foods. Some chefs add flour to fats to make a thicker sauce when sautéing foods.

Beware of fryers. Foods prepared in a deep-fat fryer can be cross-contaminated if they share the equipment with french fries or battered chicken. Also, the oils commonly used—canola or soy—are inflammatory.

When you are invited to someone's home, let your needs be known. No one wants to be embarrassed and serve food that a guest can't eat. Explain your situation well in advance; the more notice the better, so the host has time to prepare something appropriate. I find that when I get invited to someone's home, people make dishes from my books for me—and that's a HUGE compliment! Recently I went home to New Orleans so that my extended family could meet Elle, and my aunt prepared a lunch of grilled chicken, brussels sprouts, and Herbed "Potato" Salad (page 148). Or even better, let your hosts know that you have a dish that you would love to make and share with everyone!

16

Sleep

We all know how important it is to get a full night of restorative sleep. During sleep, our bodies repair damaged tissue and quell inflammation. It's why our bodies are designed to fall asleep when it's dark outside and wake up when the sun comes up over the horizon—so that we can get the recovery time that we need. This pattern of waking with the sun and sleeping when it's dark is called your *circadian rhythm,* and it affects hormone and energy levels and how well you recover from illness. In today's world, however, many things—such as traveling across time zones; using electronic devices all hours of the day and night; experiencing stress and depression; and ingesting caffeine, sugar, and alcohol—can disrupt your body's circadian rhythm and keep you from getting that much needed, healing sleep. Here are some tips to help you get the necessary sleep your body and brain need.

Start off the day by going outside. Just as you need to be in the dark at night, you also need exposure to sunlight during the day because it is a cue to your circadian rhythm that you are awake. A great way to reset your body's natural clock is to get outdoors within twenty minutes of waking. Take a walk, do some gardening, or ride a bike. Simply being exposed to daylight will help reset your sleep cycle for the day, as well as increase vitamin D production.

Limit your exposure to blue light after sunset. Fluorescent and LED light bulbs and flat-screen TVs, as well as the displays of our computers, tablets, and phones, are abundant in "blue light." This means that every time you use such light bulbs, watch TV, or look at the screens of electronic devices, the light signals to your brain that it's daytime and you should be awake. This in turn inhibits your body's natural production of melatonin, the hormone that tells your body and brain to feel sleepy and go to bed. For that reason I recommend limiting your use of artificial lighting after sundown, replacing the bulbs in your lamps to amber light bulbs, turning off all electronic devices two hours before bedtime, and sleeping in a dark, cool room. This will help retrain your body to recognize that nighttime is for sleep, while daytime is when you want to be awake and energetic.

Wear amber glasses. While minimizing your use of artificial lighting at night is a great first step, most of us can't go completely without using lights or looking at screens all evening long. That's why my favorite sleep tool, and the one that I won't travel without, is my pair of blue light–blocking or amber glasses. The amber-colored lenses in the glasses block out the blue light that reduces melatonin production so that your body naturally gets sleepy as you near bedtime. Just put them on as soon as the sun begins to set and take them off at bedtime. My favorites amber glasses can be found on my website.

If you're going to be using your computer a lot after sundown, try downloading the f.lux software, which adjusts to the time of day and creates an amber hue on your computer screen after dark. A similar app for iPhones and iPads is called Night Shift.

Go with the seasons. You're probably thinking that it's going to be difficult to power down your electronics, dim your lights, and prepare for bed in the wintertime, when it gets dark earlier. Will you be sleeping too much? Just as your body is designed to move with the day, it's also meant to move with the seasons. You will sleep more during the winter, and that's what you need. Winter is a time to conserve your energy and repair your body, especially if you live in a colder climate. As appetites change seasonally, so do sleep requirements.

Consider melatonin supplementation to support healthy sleep patterns. Your body naturally produces the sleep hormone melatonin as it becomes dark outside in order to help you fall asleep and stay asleep. However, because of our abundant use of artificial lighting, sometimes unpredictable schedules, and occasional jet lag, I often take a melatonin supplement twenty minutes before bed to ensure that I get a full night of restorative sleep if my circadian rhythm has become disrupted. I recommend a sustained-release formula, such as the one I carry in my online store, so that the melatonin is released in two waves and you are able to sleep all night long.

Relieve your stress. A huge component of getting a good night's sleep is to regularly relieve your stress so that you can peacefully drift off each night. I enjoy using the HeartMath sensor and app to synchronize my breath, heart, and mind (see Resources). As a very goal-oriented person (yes, even in my stress reduction!), I love that these tools let you set goals and track your progress. I also spend time in my infrared sauna several nights a week so that I can relieve stress and muscle tension while also detoxifying (a double win!). However, remember that the key is to find the stress-relieving activity that works for *you*—whether it's yoga, meditation, journaling, or walking in nature—and then to stick with it!

Finally, I love winding down with a hot bath using Stress-Relieving Lavender Spa Bath Salts (page 258) and drinking a cup of Gut-Soothing Collagen Tea (page 126) before bed. A hot bath helps your lymphatic system flush toxins more easily, and the amino acids in the collagen help keep your blood sugar balanced overnight, and the glycine helps to promote sleep.

17

Food Reintroduction

A key part of The Myers Way is systematically reintroducing some of the foods that you eliminated in order to determine which foods you can add back in to your diet to maximize variety, which foods you can splurge on in moderation for special occasions, and which are your "absolute no" foods that you'll permanently avoid. For example, as I mentioned at the beginning of this book, I know that as long as I'm at the healthy end of the autoimmune spectrum and feeling great, I can occasionally enjoy foods such as rice, eggs, and even a rare gluten-free, dairy-free cupcake without having a flare-up of symptoms. Then, if something such as mold exposure or a period of high stress causes me to move in the unhealthy direction on the spectrum, I cut those foods out again and go back to emphasizing the four pillars until I've worked my way back to optimal health. On the other hand, I know that gluten and dairy are "absolute no" foods for me (and anyone else with autoimmunity), so I will never add them back in.

If you have already followed the thirty-day plan in *The Autoimmune Solution* and completed the reintroduction protocol, then you know what your "yes," "in moderation," and "absolute no" foods are and you can skip this chapter. And, if you are new to The Myers Way, I highly recommend sticking with the dietary plan laid out in this book for thirty days and then following the reintroduction protocol below to determine your own lists of "yes," "in moderation," and "absolute no" foods.

Big Picture Tips for Food Reintroduction

- I do not recommend that you ever add back in gluten and cow dairy (the proteins in camel, sheep, and goat dairy are different from those in cow dairy, so you may add these in to see whether you can tolerate them; see opposite page).

- Always avoid high amounts of caffeine, sugar, alcohol, salt, grains, and legumes.

- Always avoid "toxic foods" such as artificial sweeteners, genetically modified foods, artificial colors, artificial preservatives, dyes, high-fructose corn syrup, *trans* fats, and hydrogenated fats.

- Remember that your health is a continuum. You might find that during different times in your life, you might tolerate different foods.

Potential Challenges

- If your symptoms have not resolved yet, more healing needs to be done, so this is likely not the best time to try to reintroduce foods.
  Suggestion: Follow the tips in *The Autoimmune Solution* to investigate further avenues for healing or simply give your body more time on The Myers Way.

- You may not always feel a difference in outward symptoms even if your body is becoming inflamed or reactive.
  Suggestion: Work with your doctor to measure inflammatory and/or autoimmune lab markers, for example, your thyroid antibodies, before and after food reintroductions.

- If you are on medications to suppress your immune system, you may not notice a reaction.

  Suggestion: Work with your doctor to reduce any unnecessary medications now that you have healed your gut, reduced inflammation, tamed toxins, healed infections, and relieved stress. When you've been able to get off your immunosuppressive drugs, you can begin reintroducing foods to see how your body is really responding.

Foods to Reintroduce

I recommend reintroducing the foods below in the following order to see whether you can tolerate them and add them back into your diet (however, you don't have to reintroduce any of the foods listed below; you are welcome to simply stick with The Myers Way–approved foods).

- Eggs

- Tomatoes

- Potatoes

- Eggplant

- Peppers

- Goat dairy

- Sheep dairy

If you desire, you may reintroduce the following to see whether you can tolerate them and add them back into your diet *on occasion*:

- Alcoholic drinks

- Caffeinated drinks

- Sugar

- Nuts and seeds

- Gluten-free grains

- Legumes

- Gluten- and dairy-free baked goods for special occasions

How to Reintroduce Foods

For the first seven foods listed above (eggs, tomatoes, potatoes, eggplant, peppers, goat dairy, sheep dairy), I recommend a specific protocol of "bombarding" your system with each of the foods by eating **one food at a time—three times a day for three days**. If a food is a trigger of inflammation for you, I want you to have the best chance to determine that right away, rather than allowing silent inflammation to sneak in, causing you unwanted health problems.

- Reintroduce only *one* food at a time. If you eat two foods on the same day and you have a bad reaction, you won't know which one is the culprit!

- Reintroduce a food by consuming it three times a day for three days.

- Return to The Myers Way for three days before trying the next food.

- If you have a reaction, stop eating that food and wait until you are symptom-free before you try the next food.

- If you don't have a reaction, leave that food out of your diet, spend three days on The Myers Way, and then continue to the next food.

- At the end of the food reintroduction protocol, you can add back in to your diet each food that you have tested and found to be safe.

What to Look for as You Reintroduce Foods

Look for signs of inflammation. Remember: reactions can be very mild at first and can take up to seventy-two hours to appear. Listen carefully to what your body is saying. Common symptoms to look for include

- Increase in autoimmune blood markers

- Brain fog

- Changes in inflammatory/autoimmune lab markers

- Depression/anxiety

- Changes in the bowels (diarrhea or constipation)

- Disruptions in sleep

- Fatigue

- Gas or bloating

- Headache

- Heightened emotions

- Joint pain

- Mood swings

- Rash

- Sleepiness after meals

- Swelling in hands, feet, and legs

- Weight gain

If you notice one or any combination of these symptoms, then stop eating the new food immediately. I recommend that you track your symptoms and how your body is responding by using The Myers Way Symptom Tracker (page 19). Using The Myers Way Symptom Tracker will allow you to understand which foods you can add back in to your diet, which ones you can enjoy only occasionally, and which ones are your "absolute no" foods that you should permanently avoid.

18

Supplements

The number one question I'm asked is, "Do you think everyone should take supplements?"

The simple answer is, Yes! That's because the unfortunate truth is that our modern world simply can't provide all of the essential nutrients we need for optimal health. Our Western diet is filled with nutrient-poor and calorie-dense processed foods, GMOs, and pesticides. Even our soil has become depleted of nutrients, which means that the food that's grown in it has declined in nutritional value. We are constantly exposed to toxins in our food, water, air, and even personal care and cleaning products. Our stress levels have skyrocketed, and many people are dealing with gut issues, such as Candida and SIBO, which interfere with proper nutrient absorption.

The number two question I'm asked is, "Which ones should I take?" There are four essential supplements I believe everyone should take—a comprehensive multivitamin, omega-3 fish oil, probiotics, and vitamin D with vitamin K (see pages 290–291). Xavier and I take these every day, and I have been giving them to Elle since the day she was born.

From there, you may need additional supplements depending on your unique genetic and biochemical needs, as well as your individual health conditions. As I was healing from Candida, SIBO, leaky gut, heavy metal overload, and then later toxic mold exposure, I took a lot of supplements to help me recover more rapidly. As I have healed, I have been able to reduce the number of supplements I take. Since my detox pathways are compromised and I have a predisposition to autoimmunity, I still take supplements to keep me on the healthy end of the autoimmune spectrum.

Here's an overview of the most common supplement needs that I see in my autoimmune patients.

You can find a handy list of links for all of the resources listed in this book, plus get a free $10 gift card to use in my online store on Amy Myers MD supplements and step-by-step resources, by visiting my website at amymd.io/cookbook.

The Four Essential Supplements

The Myers Way Multivitamin

A high-quality multivitamin is critical for building a strong foundation for optimal health. The Myers Way Multivitamin contains high levels of key nutrients, including premethylated B vitamins, calcium and vitamin D, vitamins A and C, and magnesium, in their most bioavailable forms. In addition, I specially designed The Myers Way Multivitamin for those people with autoimmunity and thyroid dysfunction, including Hashimoto's and Graves' diseases, and it features optimal amounts of iodine, selenium, and zinc to support immune and thyroid function.

Omega-3 Fish Oil

This supplement prevents and fights inflammation, which is the root of all chronic illness, particularly autoimmunity. Omega-3 fatty acids are also critical for brain health, memory, mood, and cognition because your brain is 60 percent fat. Finally, these fatty acids also support thyroid function by improving cell integrity so that thyroid hormones can get into your cells and attach to receptors. My recommendation is to take at least 1,000 milligrams of fish oil daily.

Probiotics

Recent research has shown there are more bacteria in us and on us than our own cells. The trillions of microorganisms that live in your digestive tract make up your gut *microbiome*. They play an enormous role in your immune system health, because nearly 80 percent of your immune system is in your gut. Taking a daily probiotic, which is a dose of the good bacteria, helps strengthen your immune system and prevent pathogenic yeast and bacteria from overgrowing. Look for a probiotic with both *Lactobacillus* and *Bifidobacterium*. I recommend taking 100 billion CFU of probiotic if you're trying to overcome any gut dysfunction such as leaky gut or Candida overgrowth and 30 billion CFU as a maintenance dose.

Vitamin D Containing Vitamin K

Vitamin D deficiency is nearly ubiquitous in the autoimmune patients I see, and studies estimate that one billion people worldwide have insufficient vitamin D levels. This is due in part to diets low in foods containing vitamin D and the fact that we spend less time exposed to sunlight, which is what triggers your body's natural production of vitamin D. For this reason, I find that most people with autoimmunity need between 1,000 and 5,000 IU of vitamin D3 daily. (I recommend that you consult with your physician and get your vitamin D levels tested if you take more than 2,000 IU a day because it is a fat-soluble vitamin and can be toxic at high doses.) It is important to make sure you take vitamin K with your vitamin D. Vitamin K increases absorption of vitamin D into bones without leading to calcium plaque buildup in your arteries.

Bonus Essentials

Methylation Support

This is a supplement that I consider an "essential" for myself or anyone else with one or more *MTHFR* (methylenetetrahydrofolate reductase) gene mutations. *MTHFR* gene mutations reduce your ability to methylate—a biochemical process that turns toxins into safer substances that can be flushed from your body. A daily methylation support supplement containing premethylated vitamin B12, vitamin B6, folate, and magnesium will help your body methylate optimally and prevent toxin buildup.

The Myers Way Paleo Protein Powder

I am not kidding when I say that I am seriously addicted to this protein powder! It makes the most delicious, creamy smoothies and is completely approved for The Myers Way because the protein comes from grass-fed, pasture-raised cows that were never given hormones, antibiotics, or GMOs. It's a perfect and convenient way to ensure that you're getting all nine of the essential amino acids that your body needs, while also enjoying a tasty treat. I recommend one scoop of The Myers Way Paleo Protein in a smoothie each day.

Supplements for Inflammation and Autoimmunity

These are the supplements that I personally take, recommend to my autoimmune patients, and are included in *The Autoimmune Solution*.

Acetyl-Glutathione

Glutathione is your body's biggest detoxifier. It helps carry toxins out of your body by binding itself to free radicals—molecules that damage your tissues. Without enough glutathione, your body cannot properly detox, which means that the toxins linger in your bloodstream longer or even get stored in fat. Studies show that people with autoimmunity and cancer have lower glutathione levels than healthy individuals. Glutathione is not well absorbed orally so you must make sure you are taking acetyl-glutathione with nanotechnology, as it is not broken down in the gut. I recommend 300–900 milligrams daily for optimal detoxification. Acetyl-glutathione works synergistically with curcumin and resveratrol.

Curcumin (Fat Soluble)

This supplement comes from the spice turmeric, which has been used medicinally for thousands of years. It helps reduce inflammation, fight free radicals, and support your detox pathways. However, you would have to eat pounds and pounds of turmeric to get all of its amazing health benefits. It is important to take a fat-soluble curcumin so that the curcumin can actually get into your cells where it acts to reduce inflammation. I recommend supplementing with 1,000 milligrams of fat-soluble curcumin each day. Curcumin works synergistically with acetyl-glutathione and resveratrol.

Resveratrol

Resveratrol is the health-supporting polyphenol found in red wine. It's a free radical scavenger that supports a balanced immune system, a healthy inflammatory response, and optimal aging. In order to take advantage of resveratrol's health benefits without all of the sugar and alcohol found in red wine, take 25 milligrams of supplemental resveratrol per day. Resveratrol works synergistically with acetyl-glutathione and curcumin.

Immune Booster

Colostrum (from humans or animals) is the first milk that comes from breastfeeding, and it is chock-full of immunoglobulins, also known as antibodies. These immunoglobulins are proteins your immune system uses to help fight off invaders, and they are the first line of defense in your gut. I find that most of my autoimmune patients are low in immunoglobulins. You can boost your immunoglobulin levels and restore your immune system and gut to optimal function by supplementing with 2 grams of immunoglobulins daily.

Supplements for Gut Health

Virtually all of my autoimmune patients are dealing with gut issues, and restoring your gut health is a crucial first step in reversing any autoimmune condition. These are the supplements I recommend for overcoming leaky gut and maintaining a healthy gut for life.

The Myers Way Collagen Protein

Collagen is the glue that holds your body together. Gram for gram it's even stronger than steel! It's rich in four key amino acids that repair the lining of your gut, in addition to supporting healthy bones and joints, cardiovascular health, and beautiful hair, skin, and nails. Be sure you are getting collagen from a grass-fed, non-GMO, hormone-free, and antibiotic-free source. Take up to 25 grams (about 2 tablespoons) of collagen peptides per day for optimal gut health. I use collagen daily in my smoothies (pages 105–113) or I drink a cup of Gut-Soothing Collagen Tea (page 126) before bed.

L-Glutamine

Because a leaky gut is a precursor to autoimmunity, I recommend that all of my autoimmune patients supplement with L-glutamine in order to maintain optimal gut health. L-glutamine is an amino acid that helps your gut cells turn over faster so that your gut lining can repair itself more quickly. I recommend 2,500–4,000 milligrams of L-glutamine daily.

RECOMMENDED SUPPLEMENTS

The Four Essentials

Supplement	Recommended Daily Dose
The Myers Way Multivitamin	6 pills
Omega-3 fish oil	1,000–2,000 mg
Probiotics	100 billion CFU for restoring gut health; 30 billion CFU for maintenance
Vitamin D with vitamin K	1,000–5,000 IU
Bonus Essentials	
Methylation support (if you have *MTHFR* gene mutations)	1–2 pills
The Myers Way Paleo Protein	1 scoop

For Inflammation and Autoimmunity

Supplement	Recommended Daily Dose
Acetyl-glutathione	300–900 mg
Curcumin (fat soluble)	1,000 mg
Resveratrol	25 mg
Immune booster	2 g

For Gut Health

Supplement	Recommended Daily Dose
The Myers Way Collagen Protein	Up to 25 g
L-Glutamine	2,500–4,000 mg
Complete enzymes	1–2 pills with each meal
Probiotics	100 billion CFU for restoring gut health; 30 billion CFU for maintenance

Complete Enzymes

Digestive enzymes help you digest and absorb the nutrients from your food, easing your digestive burden. In addition, they break down inflammatory antigens in your food in order to minimize damage to your gut, as well as helping you break down and flush gluten from your system more quickly in case you accidentally consume it. I always take digestive enzymes when I travel or eat out in a restaurant. I recommend taking 1–2 pills with each meal.

Probiotics

As I say previously ("The Four Essential Supplements"), I recommend taking 100 billion CFU of probiotic if you're trying to overcome any gut dysfunction and 30 billion CFU as a maintenance dose.

HOW TO CHOOSE QUALITY SUPPLEMENTS

Since the supplement industry is unregulated, many supplements don't contain what you need. It's important that you do your research to ensure that you aren't wasting your money. The Natural Products Association has a good manufacturing practices (GMP) certification program, which means that GMP-certified manufacturers have evaluated the purity, quality, strength, and composition of your supplement.

Also check for third-party testing—not by the manufacturer—to ensure quality and purity. You don't want fish oil that contains mercury or other toxic heavy metals because the fish a company uses for the oil are loaded with them.

Over time, supplements do lose their potency, so you want to make sure that the ones you purchase will be potent at the expiration date, not the manufacture date. You also want supplements to be shelf-stable without needing refrigeration so they can go wherever you go.

Acknowledgments

I was so excited when I was approached to write this cookbook! I have enjoyed healthy baking and cooking since my childhood, and I felt a cookbook was a key missing piece for those of us with autoimmunity. When I realized the aggressive delivery schedule for this cookbook, I freaked out. I could not imagine how I was possibly going to be able to develop and test over 150 recipes, along with seeing patients, being a mom, running my company, and being of service to my community. I quickly sought out the help of my registered dietician, Dana Faris, RD LD, and together over a weekend we created a list of recipes and a framework for this cookbook. And then she went to work, testing and retesting to ensure that each and every recipe in this book was absolutely perfect and delicious. Dana, you have been a true godsend, and I could not have completed this amazing cookbook without you. Thank you!

In addition, I would like to thank the following people.

Gideon Weil, thank you for always believing in me and my mission. You and the entire HarperOne team are a true pleasure to work with and I am so happy I was able to come back and do this project with you.

Stephanie Tade, as I have said before, you are so much more than my book agent. You are a true advocate, confidante, and friend. Thank you for going above and beyond at all times and especially with this project.

Jordyn Bean, thank you for swooping in at the end and helping me to get this book to convey my mission, my passion, and my words. Sometimes I think you know what I would say better than I do.

Tracy Behar and Little Brown, thank you for allowing me to do this cookbook with Gideon and HarperOne. I so appreciate your willingness and generosity.

Harriet Bell for your assistance in bringing this book to life.

My entire team at AmyMyersMD.com, you guys rock! I could not ask for a better group of people to work with. Thank you all for believing in me and my mission and, most important, thank you for helping me to empower so many people around the world to take back their health. I could not do it without you.

To my patients and the AmyMyersMD.com community, you are why I do what I do. Thank you for your trust and your faith in me. I appreciate each of you for your commitment to taking back your health. You inspire me.

My dear husband, Xavier, thank you for putting up with all my long work hours and for supporting me always.

My precious daughter, Elle, you are my everything. I love you.

Tia Norma and Nana, thank you both for all that you do for our family and for Elle. All the extra hours and weekend playdates with Elle so that I could work on this book. I could never do all that I do without you both.

Most important, to my mom and my dad for teaching me how to bake and cook, and for instilling in me the nourishing power of food. I love you and I miss you both.

Resources

You can find a handy list of links for all of the resources listed in this book, plus get a free $10 gift card to use in my online store on Amy Myers MD supplements and step-by-step resources, by visiting my website at amymd.io/cookbook.

Amy Myers MD Online

Connect with me online for empowering information and helpful tips.

Website: amymyersmd.com

The Myers Way Community on Facebook: amymyersmd.com/community

Facebook: www.facebook.com/amymyersmd

Twitter: @amymyersmd

Instagram: @amymyersmd

Pinterest: www.pinterest.com/amymyersmd

Amy Myers MD Books, Summits, and Programs

You can find the following resources on my website, amymyersmd.com:

The Autoimmune Solution (book)

The Thyroid Connection (book)

The Autoimmune Solution Summit

The Thyroid Connection Summit

The Myers Way Autoimmune Solution Program

The Myers Way Candida Breakthrough Program

The Myers Way SIBO Breakthrough Program

The Myers Way Leaky Gut Breakthrough Program

The Myers Way Parasite Breakthrough Program

The Myers Way Guide to the Gut eCourse

The Myers Way Elimination Diet eCourse

The Myers Way Meal Planning Tool

Working with a Functional Medicine Practitioner

Functional medicine practitioners are a great resource for identifying and addressing the root cause of your symptoms.

Amy Myers MD Wellness Coaching

My Wellness Coach is a registered dietician who works right alongside me treating patients from all over the world who are overcoming autoimmune disease, thyroid disease, gut infections, and other chronic health conditions. She can help with special diets, recommended supplements, lab testing, goal setting, and accountability; visit amymd.io/wellness.

The Institute for Functional Medicine

I did my functional medicine training through the Institute for Functional Medicine (IFM). If you are not able to make an appointment with my Wellness Coach, I suggest you check the IFM's website to locate a practitioner in your area. Functional medicine addresses the underlying causes of disease using a systems-oriented approach and engaging both patient and practitioner in a therapeutic partnership. It is an evolution in the practice of medicine that better addresses the health-care needs of the twenty-first century; visit www.ifm.org.

American Academy of Environmental Medicine

The mission of the American Academy of Environmental Medicine (AAEM) is "to promote optimal health through prevention, and safe and effective treatment of the causes of illness by supporting physicians and other professionals in serving the public through education about the interaction between humans and their environment." The AAEM is an international organization representing physicians who specialize in environmental medicine, a type of medicine that focuses on the environmental causes of poor health; visit www.aaemonline.org.

The Myers Way Autoimmune Solution Online Program

No matter where you are on the autoimmune spectrum, The Myers Way Autoimmune Solution Program gives you the tools and information you need to support your body, your health, and your sense of well-being. The program is packed with informative resources and empowering tools to put the proven program from my *New York Times* bestseller, *The Autoimmune Solution,* into practice; visit amymd.io/autoimmunity.

Healthy Eating

- **The Myers Way Meal-Planning Tool:** This is an interactive tool that allows you to browse hundreds of The Myers Way–approved recipes to build a customized weekly meal plan and personalized shopping list; visit amymd.io/mealplan.

- **Thrive Market:** Thrive Market offers the best in organic, non-GMO, paleo, gluten-free/dairy-free foods and toxin-free household goods for 25 to 50 percent less than you'll find in the grocery store; visit www.thrivemarket.com.

- **Vital Choice:** I recommend enjoying wild-caught seafood during the thirty-day protocol and beyond. Vital Choice has excellent options for low-mercury seafood, including wild-caught salmon; visit www.vitalchoice.com.

- **ButcherBox:** ButcherBox ships high-quality meats right to your door every month! The company is committed to raising high-quality 100 percent grass-fed and grass-finished beef, organic free-range chicken, and heritage breed pork—perfect for any of my protocols; visit www.butcherbox.com.

Favorite Brands

Paleo ingredients and companies have come a long way over the past few years. Here are some of my favorite brands to use in your kitchen.

- **Bragg Apple Cider Vinegar:** This vinegar is organic and made without yeast, so it's a great option for use in my recipes; visit www.bragg.com/products/bragg-organic-apple-cider-vinegar.html.

- **Desert Farms Camel Milk:** We love camel's milk in our household. In fact, Elle has never had cow dairy and solely drinks camel's milk! It is jam packed with nutrients such as vitamin B1, zinc, and selenium; visit www.desertfarms.com.

- **Nuts.com Freeze-Dried Fruit:** In this cookbook, you will find freeze-dried fruit as a topping option in recipes such as Dark Chocolate Bark (page 236). Freeze-dried fruits are lower in sugar than traditionally dried fruit and contain no added sugars overall; visit www.nuts.com.

- **Kettle & Fire Bone Broth:** While bone broth is super easy to make at home, occasionally I don't have any homemade broth on hand. Kettle & Fire is one of my go-to brands for these instances; visit www.kettleandfire.com.

- **Nutiva:** Nutiva has everything from organic coconut oil to sustainably harvested palm oil that I use in many of my recipes; visit www.nutiva.com.

- **Organic Gemini Tigernuts:** You may be asking, "What in the world is a tigernut?" Though the name makes it sound like a nut, a tigernut is actually a root vegetable packed with prebiotic fiber! Organic Gemini provides a line of tigernut-based products, including whole tigernuts, flours, and even tigernut milks that are all The Myers Way approved; visit www.organicgemini.com.

- **Otto's Naturals Cassava Flour:** Cassava flour is a great grain-free replacement in paleo baking! I like Otto's Naturals cassava flour for its versatility and quality; visit www.ottosnaturals.com.

- **Primal Palate Organic Spices:** I'm always looking for a new way to spice up my food, and Primal Palate has made that search a lot easier! Primal Palate has created a variety of organic spice blends and individual spices to make cooking easy, fun, and flavorful; visit www.primalpalate.com.

- **Siete Family Foods Tortillas and Chips:** Siete makes the best tortillas around, not to mention tortilla chips that are to die for! This Austin-based company now offers its products all over the United States and really helps me out when I am in a time crunch; visit www.sietefoods.com.

Equipping Your Kitchen

Here are some of my favorite brands and cookware to help improve your cooking and reduce your toxic burden.

Baking Equipment

- **Stainless-Steel Baking Sheets:** Most sheet pans are made out of aluminum, which can leach into your food. Stainless steel is a better alternative for your baking needs.

- **Pyrex Baking Dishes:** Pyrex glass baking dishes come in many sizes and varieties and are incredibly durable too; visit www.pyrex ware.com.

- **KitchenAid Stand Mixer:** These machines make fast work of repetitive cooking tasks like whisking together dry ingredients, pureeing root vegetables, and beating batters. Some models even have spiralizing and food processor attachments; visit www.kitchenaid.com.

Kitchen Tools

- **Glass Measuring Cups:** These are the perfect addition to your kitchen and allow you to measure hot ingredients safely without using plastic.

- **Stainless-Steel Measuring Spoons:** Stainless steel is sturdy, durable, and makes a great alternative to standard plastic measuring utensils typically used in the kitchen.

- **Meat Thermometer:** It is very important to make sure your meat is cooked thoroughly to ensure your safety and that of family and friends. The Super-Fast Thermapen by ThermoWorks reads internal temperatures in 2 to 3 seconds; visit www.thermoworks.com.

- **Knives:** One of the most important tools to have in the kitchen is a reliable chef's knife! Some quality brands I rely on are Global (www.globalcutleryusa.com), Henckels (www.zwillingonline.com), and Shun (shun.kaiusaltd.com).

Blenders, Food Processors, and Juicers

- **Vitamix Blender:** This is one of my most used purchases! It is great for making smoothies or blending up soups and sauces; visit www.vitamix.com.

- **NutriBullet Blender:** When I'm on the run, the NutriBullet comes in handy to quickly blend up a smoothie and take it with me all in one container; visit www.nutribullet.com.

- **Breville Juicer:** My favorite juicers are the ones that give you the most nutrients from your produce and also provide you with added fiber. Breville does exactly that! I prefer ones that are slow, cold-press, or masticating juicers; visit www.brevilleusa.com.

- **Cuisinart Food Processor:** For larger servings of foods such as soups that involve blending, a food processor definitely comes in handy; visit www.cuisinart.com/products/food_processors.

- **Immersion Blender:** An immersion blender, or a stick or wand blender, makes it easy to blend up dishes and is super easy to clean; visit www.cuisinart.com/products/hand_blenders.

Pressure Cookers and Slow Cookers

- **Crock-Pot Slow Cooker:** A slow cooker makes meal preparation so easy! All you have to do is throw everything in, turn it on, and let it go for a few hours. I don't know what I would do without mine; visit www.crock-pot.com.

- **Instant Pot:** This great small appliance is a jack of all trades with the ability to function as a pressure cooker, slow cooker, sauté pan, yogurt maker, and so much more; visit www.instantpot.com.

Pots and Pans

- **Le Creuset:** This company offers a wide variety of cookware and bakeware that is incredibly durable and makes nontoxic cooking simple; visit www.lecreuset.com.

- **Lodge:** I have had my Lodge cast-iron skillet forever! It is my go-to pan for toxin-free cooking. I also love Lodge grill pans for cooking meat when grilling just isn't an option; visit www.lodgemfg.com.

- **Staub:** This is another great brand for cast-iron and nontoxic cookware! Not to mention that it comes in a variety of fun colors; visit www.staubusa.com.

Taming the Toxins

- **Toxin-Free Makeup:** I get all of my makeup from Beautycounter because the company avoids using toxic chemicals such as parabens and phthalates. Plus, it tests its products for safety using rigorous standards; visit www.beautycounter.com.

- **Toxin-Free Home and Body DVD and Recipe eBook:** I have created a DVD with step-by-step instructions on how to keep your home smelling fresh, looking clean, and best of all, toxin-free! It also comes with a recipe eBook to help you easily shop for ingredients; visit amymd.io/toxinfree.

- **Aquasana Water Filter:** Filtering your water can greatly eliminate unnecessary toxins and help to support your immune system; visit www.aquasana.com.

- **HEPA Air Filter:** You can clean the air in your home with a HEPA air filter, which I have in both my home and my office. My favorite air purifiers from IQAir are designed to remove even the tiniest particles from your air, including viruses, pet dander, dust mites, air pollution, and even cigarette smoke; visit www.iqair.com.

Relieving Stress

- **HeartMath Inner Balance:** The Inner Balance app for iPhone uses an external sensor on your earlobe to help you synchronize your heart rate, breath, and mind. It's super easy to use, and it's convenient since I always have my iPhone with me; visit www.heartmath.com.

- **Muse Meditation Headband:** This tool uses seven sensors to measure whether your mind is calm or active and then translates that data into weather sounds. When you're calm, you hear peaceful weather sounds; when your mind wanders, the weather intensifies, guiding you back to a calm state; visit www.choosemuse.com.

- **Binaural Beats:** In the mid-1800s, it was discovered that when your brain receives two different frequencies, one in each ear, it creates a third frequency in an effort to synchronize them. This third frequency can be used to guide your mind into a more relaxed state that helps you disconnect from your anxiety; visit amymd.io/biaurnal.

- **Sunlighten Infrared Saunas:** Infrared saunas are an effective tool for natural healing and disease prevention. If purchasing your own sauna is not an option, you can also receive treatments from natural spas that have their own infrared saunas; visit www.sunlighten.com.

- **Amber Glasses:** Getting enough sleep is vital for your health and well-being! This is especially true for those of us who are ill and trying to regain our health. My amber glasses are a HUGE help in supporting a restful night's sleep so that you too can reap the benefits of adequate rest and maintain or take back your health; visit amymd.io/amber.

Index

ablation (killing thyroid gland), 13, 14
"absolute no" foods, 29
Acai Smoothie Bowl recipe, 99
acetyl-glutathione, 292–93, 295
acid reflux/heartburn, 17, 18, 20
acne, 17
acute inflammation. *See* inflammatory response
ADD/ADHD (attention-deficit/ hyperactivity disorder), 17
Advil, 24
Agua Fresca recipe, 131
Aïoli recipe, 197
Airbnb accommodations, 273
alcohol, 77, 285
allergies, 17
All-Purpose Cleaner recipe, 261
aluminum cookware, 80
Alzheimer's disease, 17, 80
amber glasses (blue light–blocking), 280
amino acids deficiency, 57–58
AmyMyersMD.com, 7
Amy Myers MD supplements resource, 290
anal itch, 20
anise seasoning, 76
ankylosing spondylitis, 33

Anne's Amazing Cinnamon-Raisin Cookies recipe, 228–29
antacids, 24
antibiotic-resistant "super germs," 41
antibiotics: leaky gut caused by, 24; non-organic meat containing, 41
antioxidants: carotenoids, 115; cocoa powder as source of, 45; curcumin, 63–64; flavonoids, 115, 121
anxiety, 20, 27, 287
apple cider vinegar, 66, 76, 255. *See also specific recipe*
apples: Apple-Cinnamon Compote recipe, 211; Apple Crisp recipe, 244; Apple Snacks recipe, 221; Apple-Stuffed Pork Chops with Maple Glaze recipe, 170
Apricot-Chicken Salad recipe, 146
arrowroot flour, 51, 76
arthritis, 17, 20
asparagus: Bacon-Wrapped Asparagus recipe, 182; Mushroom and Asparagus Caulisotto recipe, 179
asthma, 17
"Atlantic" salmon, 60
attention-deficit/hyperactivity disorder (ADD/ADHD), 17

author's story, 2–3, 13–15
autoimmune conditions myths, 6
autoimmune diseases: author's experience with, 2–3, 13–15; connection between gluten and, 15, 27–30; connection between pesticides and, 40, 41; conventional medicine's approach to, 15–17; Dad's story on polymyositis, 3–4; demographics in America, 5; how chronic inflammation can lead to, 17–18; The Myers Way used to treat, 17; supplements to help autoimmunity and, 292–94, 295; type of microbe and associated, 33. *See also specific condition*
The Autoimmune Solution (Myers), 2, 3, 7, 9, 42, 50, 64
The Autoimmune Solution Cookbook (Myers): batch cooking recipes of, 44; as companion to The Myers Way, 7–9; free from all toxic and inflammatory foods, 30; healing by using the recipes in, 7, 26–27, 30, 35; why this book was written, 6–7. *See also healing*
The Autoimmune Solution thirty-day protocol, 66
autoimmune spectrum: author's story on experience on the, 2–3; calculating your place on, 21–22
autoimmunity reversal myth, 6
avocado oil, 48, 49
avocados: all about, 144; Bison Chili recipe, 164; BLC Tacos recipe, 88; Five-Vegetable Guacamole recipe, 220; histamine intolerance and, 255; Mango-Avocado Salsa recipe, 210; Roasted Sweet Potato Rounds with Smoked Salmon recipe, 92; Sweet Potato-Bacon Hash with Avocado Cream recipe, 90; Tropical Nicaraguan Salad recipe, 144; Wild-Caught Shrimp Sushi Rolls recipe, 225

bacon: Bacon-Wrapped Asparagus recipe, 182; BLC Tacos recipe, 88; Chicken Rollatini with Bacon and Pesto recipe, 154; histamine intolerance and, 255; Loaded and Baked Sweet Potatoes recipe, 191; Roasted Brussels Sprouts with Bacon recipe, 187; Sweet Potato-Bacon Hash with Avocado Cream recipe, 90; Wilted Greens with Bacon recipe, 193
bacteria: antibiotic-resistant, 41; bystander activation response to, 32; molecular mimicry response to, 25, 32; reinoculating with healthy, 26; SIBO, 15, 24, 25–26, 53, 87, 227, 255, 289; type of microbe and associated disorder, 33. *See also* infections; viruses
baking powder, 44
bananas: Acai Smoothie Bowl recipe, 99; Banana Pudding recipe, 242–43; histamine intolerance and, 255; Tigernut Oatmeal recipe, 87, 98; used in smoothies, 106
basil seasoning, 76
batch cooking, 44
Bath and Sink Scrub recipe, 262
bath products. *See* toxin-free products
bay leaf seasoning, 76
beauty products: Beautycounter resource for, 257; toxin-free recipes for personal care and, 80, 258–60; travel tips on packing clean, 274
beef: all about, 55–56; Beef Jerky recipe, 224; internal temperatures for, 56. *See also specific recipe*
beef tallow, 49
beets: Bison Chili recipe, 164; Ketchup recipe, 199; No-Mato Sauce recipe, 198; Purple Perfection recipe, 115; Root Vegetable Chips recipe, 215; Root Vegetable Pancakes recipe, 186
belching/passing gas, 18, 20
Berries and Cream topping, 98

Betty's Italian Dressing, 57
Betty's Italian Dressing recipe, 205
beverages: alcoholic, 77; caffeinated, 77,
    285; healthy, 76; juices, 76, 114–18,
    248–49; other types of, 119–31;
    smoothies, 76, 99, 104–13, 248–49;
    Specific Diet Chart on, 248–49
Bifidobacterium, 26, 291
birth control pills, 24
Birthday Cupcakes recipe, 50, 234–35
Bison Chili recipe, 164
Blackberry-Basil Mule recipe, 119, 127
Blackberry Vinaigrette recipe, 207
black pepper: all about, 61–62; flavorful
    seasoning using ground, 76
blackstrap molasses, 65
BLC Tacos recipe, 88
blenders, 81
bloating: food reintroduction and
    symptom of, 287; inflammatory
    symptom of, 18; The Myers Way
    Symptom Tracker on, 20
blood clots, 17
Blueberry-Lemon Compote recipe, 211
blue light–blocking or amber
    glasses, 280
"blue light" exposure, 280
the body: food reintroduction and
    possible reactions by, 287–88;
    functional medicine's system
    approach to, 14–15; using nontoxic
    products for, 257. *See also* personal
    care recipes
bone broth. *See* Gut-Healing Bone
    Broth recipe
Bragg apple cider vinegar, 66
"brain fog," 17, 20, 287
Braised Pork Ribs recipe, 171
breakfast: all about, 87; recipes for,
    86–102; Specific Diet Chart on,
    247–48
broccoli: Creamy Vegetables "Alfredo"
    recipe, 190; Create Your Own
    Coconut Curry recipe, 174–75;
    thyroid condition and, 52

broccolini: Broccolini with Garlic and
    Lemon recipe, 192; description
    of, 192
brussels sprouts: Brussels Sprouts and
    Red Cabbage Salad recipe, 142;
    Mardi Gras Salad recipe, 143;
    Roasted Brussels Sprouts with
    Bacon recipe, 187; thyroid condition
    and, 52
bulk buying, 43–44
ButcherBox.com, 42
butternut squash: Butternut Squash-Sage
    Soup recipe, 138; Curried Carrot
    Soup recipe, 137; Mardi Gras Salad
    recipe, 143; Turkey-Butternut Squash
    Hash recipe, 89; Turkey Pot Pie
    recipe, 158–59
bystander activation, 32

cabbage, 52
cacao: cacao nibs, 44–45; flavorful
    seasoning using, 76
caffeinated drinks, 77, 285
camel's milk, 76
Campylobacter, 33, 34
cancer treatments, 15–16
Candida overgrowth, 24, 25–26, 53, 87,
    227, 289
Caramelized Banana Compote recipe, 211
Caramelized Onions recipe, 72
cardiovascular disease, 17
Carolina Pulled Pork recipe, 169
carotenoids, 115
carrots: Bison Chili recipe, 164; Carrot
    Cake topping, 98; Curried Carrot
    Soup recipe, 133, 137; Five-Vegetable
    Guacamole recipe, 220; Mississippi
    Roast recipe, 160; Purple Perfection
    recipe, 115; Root Vegetable Chips
    recipe, 215; Tangy Coleslaw recipe,
    147; Thai Meatball Soup recipe, 141;
    Vegetable Fried "Rice" recipe, 177;
    Wild-Caught Shrimp Sushi Rolls
    recipe, 225

cassava flour, 51, 76
Cassava Tortillas recipe, 100
cast-iron cookware, 79
cauliflower: Cauliflower Chowder recipe, 140; Cauliflower Rice recipe, 40, 44, 67; Cauliflower Saffron "Rice" recipe, 188; Curried Carrot Soup recipe, 137; Mardi Gras Salad recipe, 143; Mashed Cauliflower and Rutabaga recipe, 189; thyroid conditions and avoiding, 52; Vegetable Fried "Rice" recipe, 177
caulisotto: description of, 179; Mushroom and Asparagus Caulisotto recipe, 179
cayenne pepper, 62
celiac disease, 5, 16, 27, 29. See also gluten
ceramic-coated pans, 79–80
CFUs (colony-forming units), 26
Chai Smoothie recipe, 109
Chai Tea Latte (Upgraded) recipe, 123
Cherry Barbecue Sauce recipe, 200
Cherry Sunrise Smoothie recipe, 105
chicken: all about, 57; Apricot-Chicken Salad recipe, 146; BLC Tacos recipe, 88; Chicken Burrito Bowl recipe, 157; Chicken "Noodle" Soup recipe, 134; Chicken Nuggets recipe, 155; Chicken Pad Thai recipe, 156; Chicken Rollatini with Bacon and Pesto recipe, 154; Chicken Satay with "Peanut" Sauce recipe, 226; Chicken Tortilla Soup recipe, 135; dining out tip on fryers, 276; Herb Roasted Chicken recipe, 152; as inflammatory food, 77; internal temperatures for, 56; Savory Breakfast Sausage recipe, 87, 93
Chimichurri Lamb Kebobs recipe, 178
Chlamydia pneumoniae, 33
chocolate: Chocolate Coconut Butter recipe, 69; Chocolate Icing recipe, 234, 238; Chocolate Whoopie Pies recipe, 238; cocoa powder, 45, 236;

Dark Chocolate Bark recipe, 236; The Myers Way Chocolate Paleo Protein, 108
chronic fatigue syndrome, 5, 33
chronic inflammation: autoimmunity and symptoms of, 17–18; description of, 17; The Myers Way Symptom Tracker to assess, 19–22
cilantro/coriander, 76
cinnamon: Anne's Amazing Cinnamon-Raisin Cookies recipe, 228–29; Apple-Cinnamon Compote recipe, 211; Cinnamon Coconut Butter recipe, 69; Cinnamon Swirl Yogurt recipe, 70; seasoning using, 76
circadian rhythm, 279
Citrobacter, 33
CLA (conjugated linoleic acid), 55
Classic Detoxifying Green Juice recipe, 116
"Clean Fifteen": Environmental Working Group list of, 53; eventually adopt the, 43
cloves seasoning, 76
cocoa powder: Dark Chocolate Bark recipe, 236; histamine intolerance and, 255; using, 45
coconut ingredients: coconut aminos, 45, 255; coconut butter, 45–46; coconut cream, 46–47; coconut flakes, 46; coconut flour, 46, 51, 76; coconut milk, 46, 76, 100; coconut oil, 46, 48, 49; coconut palm sugar, 78; coconut sugar, 47, 64
coconut oil, 46, 48, 49
coconut recipes: Coconut Butter recipe, 40, 69; Coconut Chocolate Mousse recipe, 245; Coconut Collagen Fuel Bites recipe, 218; Coconut Milk recipe, 40, 46, 68; Coconut Milk Yogurt recipe, 40, 46, 70; Coconut Shrimp recipe, 176; Coconut Yogurt Parfaits recipe, 101
collagen protein, 26, 58, 59
colostrum, 293–94

condiments: all about seasonings and, 76; recipes for dressings, sauces, and, 196–212

conjugated linoleic acid (CLA), 55

constipation: inflammatory symptom of, 18; The Myers Way Symptom Tracker on, 20

conventional medicine: approach to treating autoimmune diseases by, 15–17; prescribing medications approach of, 14. *See also* functional medicine

cookware, 78–80

copper cookware, 80

corn-made foods, 77

cortisol hormone, 34–35

Cosmetic Ingredient Review (CIR), 257

Creamy Frozen Fruit Pops recipe, 239

Creamy Hot Chocolate recipe, 125

Creamy Vegetables "Alfredo" recipe, 190

Create Your Own Coconut Curry recipe, 174–75

creatine phosphokinase (CPK), 4

Crohn's disease, 5, 16

cruciferous vegetables: debate over, 52; Roasted Vegetable Soup recipe, 139

Crunchy Maple Granola recipe, 94

cryptic antigens ("hijacking theory"), 32

Cucumber-Seaweed Salad recipe, 149

cumin seasoning, 76

curcumin, 63–64

curcumin (fat soluble), 293, 295

Curried Carrot Soup recipe, 133, 137

Dad's story, 3–4

dairy: alternatives to, 76; molecular mimicry and, 25, 32; those to avoid, 77

Dark Chocolate Bark recipe, 236

Dark Chocolate-Cherry Smoothie recipe, 108

deamidated gluten, 28

Debra's story, 1

dehydrated fruits, 53

deodorant (Lemongrass Natural Deodorant recipe), 80, 259, 274

depression, 17, 20, 27, 287

desserts: all about, 227; recipes, 228–46; Specific Diet Chart, 254–55

detoxification, 31

DHA (omega-3 fatty acids docosahexaenoic acid), 55

diabetes type 1, 5, 16

diarrhea: inflammatory symptom of, 18; The Myers Way Symptom Tracker on, 20

digestive enzymes, 296

digestive issues: inflammatory symptoms of autoimmunity and, 18; The Myers Way Symptom Tracker on, 20; myth about autoimmunity and, 6

Dijon mustard: all about, 57; Betty's Italian Dressing, 57; Pork Tenderloin with Mustard Sauce recipe, 168

dill seasoning, 76

dining out tips, 275–77

"Dirty Dozen": avoid buying the, 43; Environmental Working Group list of, 53

dressings, sauces, and condiments: dining out tips on, 276; making healthy, 195; recipes for, 196–212; Specific Diet Chart on, 252–53

The Dr. Oz Show (TV show), 2

dry eyes, 18

ear-related symptoms, 19

E. coli, 33

eczema, 18, 20

eicosapentaenoic acid (EPA), 55

electric mixers, 81

Elle (author's daughter), 5, 46, 274, 277, 289

emotional issues: depression, 17, 20; during food reintroduction, 287; The Myers Way Symptom Tracker on, 20

enameled cast-iron cookware, 78–79

environmental factors: "blue light" exposure, 280; healing leaky gut due to, 8, 15, 23–27; myth about autoimmunity and, 6. *See also* toxins

Environmental Working Group, 43, 53

EPA (eicosapentaenoic acid), 55

Epstein-Barr virus, 33–34, 35

extra virgin olive oil, 49

family involvement strategies: beginning step by step, 269–70; for getting them on board, 267–68; getting them to appreciate nourishing foods, 268–69; pick your battles, 270–71

"farmed" fish, 60

Fasano, Alessio, 24

fast foods, 77

fatigue: conventional medicine's treatment of, 18; food reintroduction and symptom of, 287; gluten sensitivity cause of, 27; inflammatory symptom of, 18; The Myers Way Symptom Tracker on, 20. *See also* weakness/tiredness

fats and oils: avocado, 48, 49; coconut, 46, 48, 49; foods with healthy, 75; nutritional importance of, 47; olive oil, 48–49; smoke points of, 47, 49; storing, 48; those to avoid, 77; vegetable oils, 47

fibrocystic breasts, 18

fibromyalgia, 5, 33

fish sauce, 50, 255

fish. *See* seafood/fish

Five-Vegetable Guacamole, 220

flavonoids, 115, 121

flours: arrowroot, 51, 76; cassava, 51, 76; coconut, 46, 51, 76; gluten-free and grain-free, 50–52; plantain, 76; recommended, 76; sweet potato, 76; tapioca, 76; tigernut, 52, 76

food additives, 77

Food and Drug Administration (FDA), 257

food labels: listing specific organic ingredients, 40; "Made with organic," 40; "100 percent organic," 40–42, 43; "USDA organic," 40

food processors, 81–82

food reintroduction: foods that can be included in, 285–86; issues to consider for, 283–84; potential challenges and tips for, 284–85; recommendations for successful, 286; what to look for during process of, 287–88

foods: "absolute no," 29; dining out, 275–77; GMOs (genetically modified organisms), 29, 40, 55, 77; healthy fats, 75; histamine intolerance and, 255; inflammatory, 24, 77; learning to appreciate nourishing, 268–69; occasional, 78; organic nonstarchy vegetables, 74; protein-rich, 74, 274; quality proteins, 74; reintroducing, 283–88; starchy vegetables, 75; toxic, 24, 77; understanding your health and, 7. *See also* organic foods

"4R" approach: 1: remove the bad, 25–26; 2: restore the good, 26; 3: reinoculate with healthy bacteria, 26; 4: repair the gut, 26

Four Essential Supplements: The Myers Way Multivitamin, 290, 295; omega-3 fish oil, 289, 290–91; probiotics, 289, 291, 296; vitamin D with vitamin K, 292, 295

Free-Radical Fighter recipe, 117

freeze-dried fruit, 53

French Vanilla Coffee Creamer recipe, 124

frequent illness, 20

Fruit Compotes recipes, 211

fruit juices: all about, 76, 114; recipes for vegetable and, 115–18

fruits: "Clean Fifteen," 43, 53; dehydrated, 53; "Dirty Dozen," 43, 53; freeze-dried, 53; organic, 40–42, 43, 53, 75. *See also specific recipe*

fruit snacks recipes, 221
fryers. *See* chicken
Fudgy Brownies recipe, 232
functional medicine: approach to
     autoimmune diseases by, 14–15;
     seeking the root cause of
     illness, 16

gallstones, 18
garlic: flavorful seasoning using, 76;
     Garlic recipe, 73
gas: food reintroduction and symptom of,
     287; inflammatory symptom of, 18;
     The Myers Way Symptom Tracker
     on, 20
gelatin: Fudgy Brownies recipe, 232;
     Gingerbread Cake recipe, 230–31;
     shopping for, 59; Zucchini Muffins
     recipe, 97. *See also* The Myers Way
     Gelatin
genital itch/discharge, 20
Get Rid of Gluten, Grains, and Legumes
     pillar, 8, 27–30
ghee, 49
ginger: flavorful seasoning using, 76;
     shopping for, 62
Gingerbread Cake recipe, 230–31
Gingerbread Cookie Smoothie
     recipe, 112
Glass Cleaner recipe, 263
glass cookware, 79
glutathione, 292–93
gluten: connection between autoimmune
     disease and, 15, 27–30; Get Rid of
     Gluten, Grains, and Legumes pillar
     on, 8, 27–30; as inflammatory food,
     77; molecular mimicry and, 25, 32.
     See also celiac disease
gluten-free: flours, 50–52; Get Rid of
     Gluten, Grains, and Legumes pillar
     on getting, 8, 27–30; myth about
     autoimmunity and being, 6; protein
     powders, 58
gluten sensitivity, 27

GMO-laden cattle feed, 54, 59
GMOs (genetically modified organisms)
     foods, 29, 40, 55, 77
goitrogens, 52
Golden Milk recipe, 120
grain-free flours, 50–52
grains: Get Rid of Gluten, Grains, and
     Legumes pillar on, 8, 27–30; as
     inflammatory food, 77
grapeseed oil, 49
Graves' disease, 5, 13–15, 16, 25,
     33–34, 58
Green Goddess Dressing recipe, 209
Grilled Bok Choy recipe, 194
ground black pepper, 61–62, 76
Guaraní people, 65–66
Guillain-Barré syndrome, 33, 34
Gut-Healing Bone Broth recipe, 40, 44,
     58, 71, 133. *See also specific recipe*
gut health: Get Rid of Gluten, Grains,
     and Legumes pillar for, 8, 27–30;
     Heal Your Gut pillar for, 8, 23–27;
     myth about autoimmunity and, 6;
     supplements to support, 294, 295;
     Tame the Toxins for, 8, 30–34, 42,
     78, 257. *See also* leaky gut
Gut-Soothing Collagen Tea recipe, 59,
     126, 281, 294

hair loss, 18
Halibut Piccata recipe, 167
Hashimoto's disease, 5, 15, 16, 25, 33
headaches: food reintroduction and
     symptom of, 287; inflammatory
     symptom of, 18; The Myers Way
     Symptom Tracker on, 20
healing: Heal Your Infections and
     Relieve Your Stress pillar for, 8, 34–
     35; inflammatory response as help
     in, 17; The Myers Way for radical,
     2, 34. *See also The Autoimmune
     Solution Cookbook* (Myers)
healthy bacteria reinoculation, 26
Heal Your Gut pillar, 8, 23–27

heartburn/indigestion, 17, 18, 20
heart-related symptoms, 19
Herbed "Potato" Salad recipe, 148
Herbed Vinaigrette recipe, 208
Herb Roasted Chicken recipe, 152
herbs, 53–54. *See also* spices
histamine intolerance, 255
home nontoxic products, 257–63
honey, 65, 78
Honey-Ginger Glazed Salmon
    recipe, 172
hormones: cortisol, 34–35; in non-
    organic meat, 41
hot baths, 281
hot chocolate: Creamy Hot Chocolate
    recipe, 125; Peppermint Hot
    Chocolate recipe, 121
household cleaners: All-Purpose
    Cleaner recipe, 261; Bath and Sink
    Scrub recipe, 262; Glass Cleaner
    recipe, 263
hydration, 274
hydrochloric acid (HCl), 26
hyperactivity, 20

illness (frequent), 20
illnesses (small intestinal bacterial
    overgrowth), 15, 24, 25–26, 53, 87
immune booster supplement, 293–94, 295
immune system: antibiotic-resistant
    "super germs" attacking, 41;
    autoimmune diseases that attack
    the, 15; bystander activation
    response of, 32; convention medicine
    on autoimmune disease and, 15–16;
    cortisol hormone impact on the,
    34–35; cryptic antigens ("hijacking
    theory") and, 32; harsh medications
    that depress the, 16; how leaky gut
    impacts the, 25; how toxins affect
    the, 30–31; inflammatory response
    of the, 17–22; molecular mimicry
    response of, 25, 32; The Myers Way
    to heal and support your, 34; The

Myers Way to support the, 57; myth
    about inability to improve, 6
immunoglobulins, 293–94, 295
indigestion, inflammatory symptom
    of, 18
infections: Candida overgrowth, 24, 25–
    26, 53, 87, 227, 289; chronic illnesses
    due to, 15; Heal Your Infections and
    Relieve Your Stress pillar, 8, 34–35;
    The Myers Way Symptom Tracker
    on, 20; SIBO, 15, 24, 25–26, 53, 87,
    227, 255, 289; supplement protocols
    for beating, 26. *See also* bacteria;
    viruses
infertility, 18
inflammatory foods, 24, 77
inflammatory response: chronic, 17;
    description of the, 17; how stress
    produces the, 34–35
inflammatory symptoms: autoimmunity
    and, 17–18; curcumin antioxidant
    to reduce, 63–64; The Myers
    Way Symptom Tracker, 19–22;
    supplements to improve, 292–94, 295
instant pots, 82
intestinal/stomach pain or cramps:
    autoimmune symptom of, 20; gas or
    bloating, 18, 20, 287; SIBO, 15, 24,
    25–26, 53, 87, 227, 255, 289
iPhones/iPads Night Shift app, 280
irritability, 20

joint pain: food reintroduction and
    symptom of, 287; inflammatory
    symptom of, 18; The Myers Way
    Symptom Tracker, 20
juicers, 81
juices: all about, 76, 114; recipes for,
    115–18; Specific Diet Chart on,
    248–49

kale: Chicken Rollatini with Bacon
    and Pesto recipe, 154; Classic

Detoxifying Green Juice recipe, 116; Five-Vegetable Guacamole, 220; Kale-Mint-Lemongrass Smoothie recipe, 108; organic nonstarchy vegetable, 74; Pesto Pizza recipe, 166; Savory Breakfast Sausage recipe, 87, 93; Turkey-Butternut Squash Hash recipe, 89; Turkey Pot Pie recipe, 158–59; Winter Salad with Maple Vinaigrette recipe, 145, 153; Zucchini Noodles with Spinach-Kale Pesto recipe, 184

Ketchup recipe, 199

kitchen: small appliances to have in your, 81–82; stocking ingredients in your, 8, 39–66; tools to have in your, 78–84

kitchen ingredient guide: baking powder, 44; cacao and cocoa, 44–45; coconut, 45–47; fats and oils, 47–50; fish sauce, 50; flours (gluten-free and grain-free), 50–52; herbs, 53–54; meat and poultry, 54–57; mustard, 57; organic fruits and vegetables, 40–42, 43, 52–53; protein powders, collagen protein, and gelatin, 57–59; recommendations when shopping for, 43–44; seafood, 59–61; seaweed, 61; spices, 61–64; sweeteners, 64–66; this book used as a, 8, 39–40; vinegar, 66

kitchen tools and equipment, information on healthy-eating supportive, 8

Klebsiella, 33, 34

knives, 82–83

Lactobacillus, 26, 291

lamb: all about, 56; Chimichurri Lamb Kebobs recipe, 178; internal temperatures for, 56; Lamb Chops with Cherry Glaze recipe, 165; Lamb Meatballs in Lettuce Wraps recipe, 173

lard, 49

Lavender Spa Bath Salts recipe, 258, 281

leaky gut: chronic illnesses due to, 15; "4R" approach to repairing, 25–26; Heal Your Gut pillar to heal a, 8, 23–27; top causes of, 24. *See also* gut health

lectins, 28–29

legumes: ditching, 28–29; Get Rid of Gluten, Grains, and Legumes pillar on, 8, 27–30; as inflammatory food, 77

Lemon Bars recipe, 233

lemongrass: Kale-Mint-Lemongrass Smoothie recipe, 108; Lemongrass Natural Deodorant recipe, 80, 259, 274; Lemongrass Natural Toothpaste recipe, 80; shopping for, 62–63

lethargy, 20

L-glutamine, 294, 295

Loaded and Baked Sweet Potatoes recipe, 191

lung-related symptoms, 19

lupus, 5, 33

"Made with organic" food label, 40

main courses: all about, 151; recipes, 152–79; Specific Diet Chart on, 250–52

mandoline, 83

Mango-Avocado Salsa recipe, 210

Maple-Cinnamon Icing recipe, 234

maple syrup, 65, 78

Mardi Gras Salad recipe, 143

Mashed Cauliflower and Rutabaga recipe, 189

meals: batch cook your, 44; recommendations when shopping and preparing, 43–44; travel tips on, 273. *See also* recipes

Mean Green Smoothie recipe, 107

Meatballs recipe, 163

Meat Marinade recipe, 202

meats: all about, 54–57; antibiotics and hormones in non-organic, 41; avoid processed, 77; ButcherBox.com for, 42; GMO-laden feed, 54, 59; GMOs (genetically modified organisms), 29, 40, 55, 77; internal temperatures for, 56. *See also specific recipes*

meat thermometers, 84

medications: conventional medicine's use of, 14; depressing the immune system, 16; leaky gut caused by some, 24; myths about autoimmunity and, 6; propylthiouracil (PTU), 13–14

medicine: conventional, 14, 15–16; functional, 14–15

melatonin, 281

methotrexate, 3

methylation supplement, 292

milk: alternatives to, 76; coconut, 46, 76, 100; Coconut Milk recipe, 40, 46, 68; Golden Milk recipe, 120

Mint-Chocolate Chip Smoothie recipe, 111

mint seasoning, 76

Mississippi Roast recipe, 160

Mixed Berry Snacks recipe, 221

mocktails, as beverage to enjoy, 76

molasses, 65, 78

molecular mimicry, 25, 32

Monterey Bay Aquarium Seafood Watch, 60–61

mood swings, 20, 287

Motrin, 24

mouth-related symptoms, 19

MSG, 50

MTHFR (methylenetetrahydrofolate reductase), 292

multiple sclerosis (MS), 5, 15, 33, 34

multivitamin, 289, 290, 295

muscle pain/aches, 18, 20

muscle stiffness, 20

mushrooms: Chicken Burrito Bowl recipe, 157; as food to enjoy, 74; Mushroom and Asparagus Caulisotto recipe, 179; Turkey Pot Pie recipe, 158–59

mustard. *See* Dijon mustard

mycophenolate mofetil (CellCept), 3

The Myers Way: *The Autoimmune Solution Cookbook* as companion to, 7–9; Dad's positive experience with, 4; four pillars of, 8, 23–35; immune system support by, 57; maintaining lifelong health through, 6; moving toward being symptom-free with, 3; online access to the six-week program called, 7; radical healing by using, 2, 34; treating autoimmune diseases using, 17

The Myers Way Chocolate Paleo Protein, 108

The Myers Way Collagen Protein, 26, 59, 104, 274, 294, 295. *See also specific recipe*

The Myers Way for Life strategies: dining out, 275–77; by getting the whole family on board, 267–71; reintroducing foods to maximize variety, 283–88; restorative sleep, 279–81; supplements, 289–96; travel tips, 273–74

The Myers Way Gelatin, 59, 96, 230, 232. *See also* gelatin

The Myers Way Multivitamin, 290, 295

The Myers Way Paleo Protein, 58, 104, 292, 295. *See also specific recipe*

The Myers Way pillars: 1: Heal Your Gut, 8, 23–27; 2: Get Rid of Gluten, Grains, and Legumes, 8, 27–30; 3: Tame the Toxins, 8, 30–34, 42, 78, 257; 4: Heal Your Infections and Relieve Your Stress, 8, 34–35

The Myers Way Symptom Tracker: assessing inflammatory symptoms using, 19–21; calculating your place on the autoimmune spectrum, 21–22

Myers Way Symptom Tracker, description and function of the, 8

The Myers Way Vanilla Paleo
Protein, 98

nausea/vomiting, 20
nervousness, 20
nightshades, 77
Night Shift app, 280
No-Mato Sauce recipe, 198
non-celiac gluten sensitivity, 27
nonstick cookware, 80
nose-related symptoms, 19
NSAIDs (nonsteroidal anti-inflammatory
    drugs), 24
nutmeg seasoning, 76
nuts, 77. See also peanuts

obesity: inflammatory symptom of, 18;
    The Myers Way Symptom Tracker
    on, 20
occasional foods, 78
oils. See fats and oils
olive oil: dining out tip on using, 276;
    shopping and selecting, 48–49;
    smoke point, 49
omega-3 fatty acids docosahexaenoic acid
    (DHA), 55
omega-3 fish oil, 289, 290–91
"100 percent organic" food label,
    40–42, 43
Onions recipe, 72
oregano seasoning, 76
organic foods: four different types
    of labels for, 40–42, 43; fruits,
    40–42, 43, 53, 75; high nutrition of,
    41–42; how to buy, 53; nonstarchy
    vegetables, 74. See also foods
Organic Green Margarita Juice
    recipe, 118

palm oil, 49
palm shortening, 50

pancakes: Pumpkin Pancakes recipe, 96;
    Root Vegetable Pancakes recipe, 186
pancreatitis, 18
parasites, 24
parsley seasoning, 76
parsnips: Curried Carrot Soup, 137;
    Herbed "Potato" Salad, 148; Mashed
    Cauliflower and Rutabaga recipe,
    189; Roasted Vegetables recipe, 183;
    Root Vegetable Chips recipe, 215;
    Root Vegetable Pancakes recipe,
    186; as starchy vegetable, 75; Sweet
    Potato Fries recipe, 185
peanuts: Chicken Satay with "Peanut"
    Sauce recipe, 226; inflammatory
    food, 77; "Peanut Butter" Cups
    recipe, 246; "Peanut" sauce recipe,
    201. See also nuts
pepper (black and white), 61–62
Peppermint Coconut Butter recipe, 69
Peppermint Hot Chocolate recipe, 121
The Perfect Fast Man Burgers recipe, 162
personal care recipes: Lemongrass
    Natural Deodorant, 80, 259, 274;
    Lemongrass Natural Toothpaste, 80;
    Stress-Relieving Lavender Spa Bath
    Salts, 258; Toothpaste, 260. See also
    the body
pesticides, 40, 41
pesto: Chicken Rollatini with Bacon and
    Pesto recipe, 154; Pesto Pizza recipe,
    166; Spinach-Kale Pesto recipe, 196;
    Zucchini Noodles with Spinach-
    Kale Pesto recipe, 184
plantain flour, 76
polymer fume fever, 80
polymyositis, 3–4
pork: all about, 56–57; Apple-Stuffed
    Pork Chops with Maple Glaze
    recipe, 170; Braised Pork Ribs recipe,
    171; Carolina Pulled Pork recipe,
    169; internal temperatures for, 56;
    Pork Tenderloin with Mustard Sauce
    recipe, 168

Porphyromonas, 33

poultry. *See* chicken; turkey

prednisone, 3

prevention: eating organic foods as, 42; toxin-taming by, 31, 42

probiotics, 289, 291, 296

produce, organic, 41–42

prolamin, 29

propylthiouracil (PTU), 13–14

protein powders: collagen, 26, 58, 59; The Myers Way Chocolate Paleo Protein, 108; The Myers Way Collagen Protein, 26, 59, 104, 274, 294, 295; The Myers Way Paleo Protein, 58, 104, 292; The Myers Way Vanilla Paleo Protein, 98. *See also specific recipe*

protein-rich foods, 74, 274

Proteus, 33

psoriasis, 5

PTFE (polyterrafluoroethylene), 80

pumpkin: Pumpkin Pancakes recipe, 96; Pumpkin Pie Smoothie recipe, 113; Pumpkin Spice Latte (Upgraded) recipe, 122; Pumpkin Spice Latte recipe, 119; Pumpkin Spice recipe, 69

Pumpkin Pie recipe, 240–41

Purple Perfection recipe, 115

quality of life myth, 6

raisins: Anne's Amazing Cinnamon-Raisin Cookies recipe, 228–29; organic fruit, 75

Ranch Dressing recipe, 206

rash, 287

Raspberry Cheesecake Bites recipe, 237

Raspberry-Lemon Snacks recipe, 221

recipes: beverages, 76, 77, 114–31, 248–49; breakfast, 87–102, 247–48; desserts, 228–46, 254–55; dressings, sauces, and condiments, 196–212, 252–53; juices, 115–18, 248–49; main courses, 151–79, 250–62; personal care, 258–63; salads, 141–49, 249–50; side dishes, 182–94, 252; smoothies, 99, 105–13, 248–49; snacks, 214–26, 253–54; soups, 134–41, 249–50; stable, 67–73, 247. *See also* meals

Red Boat (fish sauce), 50

restaurant dining, 275–77

restlessness, 20

Resveratrol, 293, 295

rheumatic fever, 33

rheumatoid arthritis, 5, 15, 16, 33

Roasted Brussels Sprouts with Bacon recipe, 187

Roasted Sweet Potato Rounds with Smoked Salmon recipe, 92

Roasted Vegetable Soup recipe, 133, 139

Roasted Vegetables recipe, 182

Root Vegetable Chips recipe, 215

Root Vegetable Pancakes recipe, 186

Rosemary-Lemon Spritzer recipe, 129

Rosemary-Sea Salt Crackers, 222

rosemary seasoning, 76

rutabagas: Herbed "Potato" Salad recipe, 148; Mississippi Roast recipe, 160; Rutabaga "Hummus" recipe, 217; as starchy vegetable, 75

saffron: Cauliflower Saffron "Rice" recipe, 188; description of, 188

salads: all about, 133; recipes, 142–49; Specific Diet Chart on, 249–50

salmon: Honey-Ginger Glazed Salmon recipe, 172; Roasted Sweet Potato Rounds with Smoked Salmon recipe, 92; shopping for, 60. *See also* seafood/fish

Sangria recipe, 130

sauces. *See* dressings, sauces, and condiments

sausage: Savory Breakfast Sausage recipe, 87, 93; Sweet Apple Breakfast Sausage recipe, 93

Savory Breakfast Sausage recipe, 87, 93

scleroderma, 5

seafood/fish: all about, 59–64; Halibut Piccata recipe, 167; overfishing, pollution, and climate change impact on, 60–61; shellfish and histamine intolerance, 255; shopping for the best, 60–61; Vitalchoice. com to buy, 42; "wild" vs. "farmed," 59–60. *See also* salmon; shrimp

sea salt, 63, 76

seasonal sleep patterns, 280–81

seasonings and condiments, 76

seaweed: all about, 61; Cucumber-Seaweed Salad recipe, 149

seeds (inflammatory food), 77

sheet pans, 83–84

shopping: avoid "Dirty Dozen," 43; buy "Clean Fifteen," 43; buy in bulk, 43–44; "100 percent organic," 40–42, 43

shrimp: Coconut Shrimp recipe, 176; shopping for, 60; Wild-Caught Shrimp Sushi Rolls recipe, 225. *See also* seafood/fish

SIBO (small intestinal bacterial overgrowth), 15, 24, 25–26, 53, 87, 227, 255, 289

side dishes: all about, 181; dining out tips on, 276; recipes, 182–94; Specific Diet Chart on, 252

skin-related symptoms, 18, 20

sleep patterns: autoimmune conditions and impact on, 18; circadian rhythm and, 279; food reintroduction and disruption in, 287; melatonin supplementation to support healthy, 281; things that can disrupt your, 279; tips for improving, 279–81

slow cookers, 82

smoke points: coconut oil, 46; fats and oils listed, 47, 49

smoothies: all about, 104; as beverage to enjoy, 76; recipes for, 99, 105–13; Specific Diet Chart on, 248–49; using bananas in, 106

snacks: all about, 213; recipes for, 214–26; Specific Diet Chart on, 253–54; travel tips on, 273

Soft Onions recipe, 72

soups: all about, 133; recipes, 134–41; Specific Diet Chart on, 249–50

soy foods, 77

Spaghetti Squash Hash Browns recipe, 91

Specific Diet Chart, 247–55

spices: all about, 61–64; ginger, 62; lemongrass, 62–63; pepper, 62; sea salt, 63; turmeric, 63–64. *See also* herbs; *specific recipe*

spinach: Apple-Stuffed Pork Chops with Maple Glaze recipe, 170; Cherry Sunrise Smoothie recipe, 105; Chicken Rollatini with Bacon and Pesto recipe, 154; Classic Detoxifying Green Juice recipe, 116; Creamy Vegetables "Alfredo" recipe, 190; Free-Radical Fighter recipe, 117; histamine intolerance and, 255; Mean Green Smoothie recipe, 107; Mint-Chocolate Chip Smoothie recipe, 111; Mushroom and Asparagus Caulisotto recipe, 179; Organic Green Margarita Juice recipe, 118; organic nonstarchy vegetable, 74; Pesto Pizza recipe, 166; Spinach-Artichoke Dip recipe, 223; Spinach-Kale Pesto recipe, 196; Tropical Green Smoothie recipe, 107; Turkey-Butternut Squash Hash recipe, 89; Wild-Caught Shrimp Sushi Rolls recipe, 225; Wilted Greens with Bacon recipe, 193; Zucchini Noodles with Spinach-Kale Pesto recipe, 184

spiralizers, 83

Splash of Sunshine recipe, 115
stable recipes: listed, 67–73; Specific Diet
    Chart on, 247
stainless-steel cookware, 79
starchy vegetables, 75
steroids, 24
stevia, 65–66, 76
Stevia rebaudiana plant, 65
stomach/intestinal pain or cramps, 20
strawberries: histamine intolerance
    and, 255; Strawberry Cheesecake
    Smoothie recipe, 110; Strawberry
    Icing recipe, 234; Strawberry Mojito
    recipe, 128
Streptococcus pyogenes, 33
stress: blamed for autoimmune
    symptoms, 13; inflammatory
    response produced by, 34–35
stress-relieving strategies: Heal Your
    Infections and Relieve Your Stress
    pillar, 8, 34–35; Stress-Relieving
    Lavender Spa Bath Salts recipe, 258,
    281; techniques and, 35, 281
sugar. *See* sweeteners
supplement essentials: MTHFR
    (methylenetetrahydrofolate
    reductase), 292; The Myers Way
    Multivitamin, 290, 295; The Myers
    Way Paleo Protein, 58, 104, 292,
    295; omega-3 fish oil, 289, 290–91;
    probiotics, 289, 291, 296; vitamin D
    with vitamin K, 292, 295
supplements: Amy Myers MD
    supplements resource on, 290;
    for beating infections, 26; for gut
    health, 294, 295; how to choose
    quality, 296; for inflammation
    and autoimmunity, 292–94; issues
    to consider for taking, 289–90;
    melatonin, 281; The Myers Way
    Collagen Protein, 26, 59, 104, 274;
    recommended, 290–96; travel tips
    on, 274
Sweet-and-Salty Trail Mix recipe, 214

Sweet Apple Breakfast Sausage
    recipe, 93
sweeteners: all about, 64; coconut sugar,
    47, 64; honey, 65, 78; maple syrup,
    65, 78; molasses, 65, 78; stevia,
    65–66
sweet potatoes: BLC Tacos recipe, 88;
    Curried Carrot Soup recipe, 137;
    Herbed "Potato" Salad, 148; Loaded
    and Baked Sweet Potatoes recipe,
    191; Roasted Sweet Potato Rounds
    with Smoked Salmon recipe, 92;
    Root Vegetable Chips recipe, 215;
    Root Vegetable Pancakes recipe,
    186; Sweet Potato-Bacon Hash with
    Avocado Cream recipe, 90; Sweet
    Potato Biscuits recipe, 102; Sweet
    Potato Fries recipe, 185
sweet potato flour, 76
swelling in hands, feet, and legs, 287

Tame the Toxins pillar, 8, 30–34, 42,
    78, 257
Tangy Coleslaw recipe, 147
Tapenade recipe, 212
tapioca flour, 76
tarragon seasoning, 76
teas: Chai Tea Latte (Upgraded) recipe,
    123; Gut-Soothing Collagen
    Tea recipe, 126; herbal and
    caffeine-free, 76
Teflon cookware, 80
Tellicherry peppercorns, 61
Thai Meatball Soup recipe, 141
throat-related symptoms, 19
thyme seasoning, 76
thyroid conditions: avoiding cruciferous
    vegetables, 52; connection between
    gluten and, 15; Graves' disease,
    5, 13–15, 16, 25, 33–34, 58;
    Hashimoto's disease, 5, 15, 16,
    25, 33
The Thyroid Connection (Myers), 2

thyroid gland: ablation (killing) the, 13, 14; goitrogens reducing function of, 52
Tigernut Butter recipe, 219
tigernut flour, 52, 76
tigernut milk, 76
Tigernut Oatmeal recipe, 87, 98
Tigernut Waffles recipe, 95
Toasted Coconut Butter recipe, 69
toasted sesame oil, 49
toothpaste: Lemongrass Natural Toothpaste recipe for, 80; recipe for, 260
toxic cookware, 79–80
toxic foods, 77
toxin-free products: Beautycounter resource for, 257; household cleaners, 261–63; personal care recipes for, 80, 258–60; travel tips on packing, 274
toxins: *The Autoimmune Solution Cookbook* recipes free from, 30; chronic illnesses due to, 15; description and danger of, 30–31; importance to switch to nontoxic products, 257; The Myers Way helping your liver to mobilize, 31; Tame the Toxins pillar, 8, 30–34, 42, 78, 257. *See also* environmental factors
toxin-taming strategies: detoxification, 31; prevention, 31
trans fats, 77
Translucent Onions recipe, 72
travel tips, 273–74
Tropical Green Smoothie recipe, 107
Tropical Nicaraguan Salad recipe, 144
Tropical Tigernut Oats topping, 98
turkey: all about, 57; internal temperatures for, 56; Savory Breakfast Sausage recipe, 87, 93; Turkey-Butternut Squash Hash recipe, 89; Turkey Pot Pie recipe, 158–59
turmeric, 63–64, 76

turnips: Herbed "Potato" Salad recipe, 148; Mississippi Roast recipe, 160; as organic nonstarchy vegetable, 75; Plantain Chips, 216; Root Vegetable Chips, 215
Tzatziki recipe, 204

ulcerative colitis, 5, 16
USDA organic food label, 40
uterine fibroids, 18

vanilla: flavorful seasoning using, 76; The Myers Way Vanilla Paleo Protein, 98; Vanilla Coconut Yogurt recipe, 70
Vegetable Fried "Rice" recipe, 177
vegetable juices: all about, 76, 114; recipes for fruit and, 115–18
vegetable oils, 47
vegetables: as beverage to enjoy, 76; "Clean Fifteen," 43; cruciferous, 52, 139; "Dirty Dozen," 43; organic, 40–42, 43, 53; organic nonstarchy, 74; starchy, 75. *See also specific recipe*
Very Berry Smoothie recipe, 106
vinegars (apple cider), 66, 76
viruses: bystander activation response to, 32; cryptic antigens ("hijacking theory") response to, 32; Epstein-Barr, 33–34, 35; molecular mimicry response to, 25, 32. *See also* bacteria; infections
Vitalchoice.com, 42
vitamin A, 47
vitamin B6, 65
vitamin B12 deficiency, 18
vitamin C, 58
vitamin D, 47, 279, 289, 291, 295
vitamin D with vitamin K, 292, 295
vitamin E, 47
vitamin K, 47, 289, 291, 295
vomiting/nausea, 20

waffles (Tigernut Waffles recipe), 95
water consumption: filtered or sparkling, 76; staying hydrated, 274
weakness/tiredness, 20. *See also* fatigue
weight issues: food reintroduction and possible, 287; inflammatory symptom of, 18; The Myers Way Symptom Tracker on, 20
white pepper, 61–62
Wild-Caught Shrimp Sushi Rolls recipe, 225
"wild" fish, 59–60
Wilted Greens with Bacon recipe, 193
Winter Salad with Maple Vinaigrette recipe, 145, 153
World's Best Asian Flank Steak recipe, 161
The World's Best Asian Marinade recipe, 203

Xavier (author's husband), 2, 3, 4, 5, 202, 203, 216, 274, 289

yeast, 66
Yersinia, 33, 34
yogurt cream, 76

zonulin protein, 24
zucchini: Chimichurri Lamb Kebobs recipe, 178; Creamy Zucchini-Basil Soup recipe, 136; Five-Vegetable Guacamole recipe, 220; Meatballs recipe, 163; Vegetable Fried "Rice" recipe, 177; Zucchini Muffins recipe, 97; Zucchini Noodles with Spinach-Kale Pesto recipe, 184

About the Author

Amy Myers, MD, is the *New York Times* bestselling author of *The Autoimmune Solution* and *The Thyroid Connection*. She is also the founder and medical director of Austin UltraHealth, a world-renowned functional medicine clinic.

During medical school, Dr. Myers developed an autoimmune thyroid condition, and after conventional medicine failed her, it became her mission to not let it fail you too. She set out to empower people to reverse autoimmunity by addressing its root causes using proven, natural solutions.

Since then, she has successfully helped thousands of patients from around the world reverse their conditions, and empowered tens of thousands more with her books, online programs, and website.

Dr. Myers lives in Austin, Texas, with her husband and their daughter, Elle, and their dog, Mocha. Their entire family lives The Myers Way, and they love introducing their family and friends to delicious meals that support optimal health.

You can find empowering resources and tips from Dr. Myers on her website at AmyMyersMD.com.